Haemoprotozoan Parasitic Diseases of Animals

The Editors

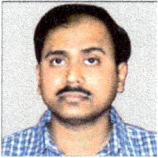

Dr. Pinaki Prasad Sengupta, is at present Principal Scientist at ICAR-NIVEDI, Yelahanka, Bengaluru. He did his B.V.Sc. and A.H. from Bidhan Chandra Krishi Viswavidyalaya, Mohanpur, Nadia, West Bengal, M.V.Sc. from same university with specialization in Veterinary Parasitology. Later he did Ph.D. (Veterinary Parasitology) from Indian Veterinary Research Institute (IVRI), Izatnagar (UP). He served in various capacities in his scientific carrier at IVRI, Izatnagar (UP), National Research Centre on Equines, Hisar before joining NIVEDI (formerly PD_ADMAS) during 2002. He has led many prestigious research projects funded by ICAR, DBT and NATP in his career. He has more than 40 publications and two patents to his credit till date. He has also got a number of awards and fellowships for his professional excellence. He has vast experience in working on hemaoprotozoan diseases including theileriosis, babesiosis and trypanosomosis.

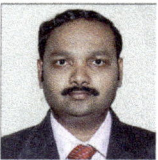

Dr. Paramanandham Krishnamoorthy did his B.V.Sc. and M.V.Sc. in Veterinary Pathology from Madras Veterinary College, Tamilnadu Veterinary and Animal Sciences University, Chennai and did his Ph. D from Veterinary College, Karnataka Veterinary, Animal and Fisheries Sciences University, Bengaluru. He is currently holding the post of Scientist at ICAR-National Institute of Veterinary Epidemiology and Disease Informatics, Bengaluru. He has worked as Assistant Professor, Apollo College of Veterinary Medicine, Jaipur and Veterinary Surgeon, Dr.ALM Post graduate Institute of Basic Medical Sciences, University of Madras. He has specialized in epidemiology, nutritional pathology, molecular biology and laboratory animal management. Dr. Krishnamoorthy is a recipient, as member of team got ICAR Outstanding Team Research Award during 2010 and Fellow of Academy of Sciences for Animal Welfare (FASAW). He has 60 research papers apart from book, book chapters, bulletins, training manuals, *etc.*, He handled seven Institute funded projects and working on spatio-temporal, GIS based analysis and field epidemiology of livestock diseases in India.

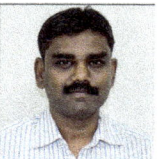

Dr. Mohandoss Nagalingam has obtained B.V.Sc., degree from Veterinary College and Research Institute, Namakkal, under Tamilnadu Veterinary and Animal Sciences University, Chennai and M.V.Sc., from G. B. Pant University of Agriculture and Technology, Pantnagar. He is working as Scientist in ICAR- National Institute of Veterinary Epidemiology and Disease Informatics, Bengaluru. He has worked as Veterinary Assistant Surgeon in Animal Husbandry Department, Tamilnadu for about seven years. He has 13 research publications in the peer reviewed journals along with book, book chapters, bulletins, manuals, *etc.* He has handled institute and DBT research projects. He is involved in development of diagnostics.

Haemoprotozoan Parasitic Diseases of Animals

– Editors –

P.P. Sengupta

P. Krishnamoorthy

M. Nagalingam

2018

Daya Publishing House®

A Division of

Astral International Pvt. Ltd.

New Delhi – 110 002

ISBN: 9789387057647 (Internatinal Edition)

Publisher's Note:

Published by : **Daya Publishing House®**
A Division of
Astral International Pvt. Ltd.
– ISO 9001:2015 Certified Company –
4736/23, Ansari Road, Darya Ganj
New Delhi-110 002
Ph. 011-43549197, 23278134
E-mail: info@astralint.com
Website: www.astralint.com

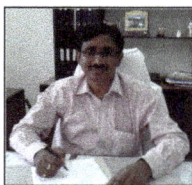

Dr. Parimal Roy

Director,

Indian Council of Agricultural Research (ICAR)
- National Institute of Veterinary Epidemiology
and Disease Informatics (NIVEDI),
Post Box No.6450, Yelahanka,
Bengaluru 560064, Karnataka

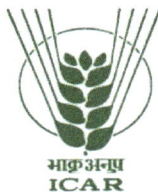

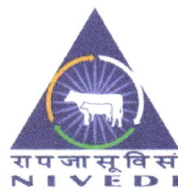

Foreword

I am very much pleased to know that the lecture notes of training course on "Epidemiology, diagnosis and control of the haemoprotozoan parasitic diseases" during 10th to 19th January, 2014, is going to be published in the form of book. The vector borne haemoprotozoan parasites in animals are major concerned in economic losses due to animal diseases. In spite of the modern system of management, these diseases are very much prevailing in our livestock sector causing severe reduction in animal production.

Today, the field veterinarians are facing new challenges to control parasites in the wake of drug resistance, diagnosis of subclinical infections, vector control and vaccine development. The emergence of transboundary parasitic diseases and their vectors in new geographical areas is augmented by globalization of trade, transport of animals between countries, changing climate and tourism. These infections pose a serious threat to our socio-economic development. The importance of controlling such infections is most required. Therefore, I strongly believe that this book will be very useful and informative to the farmers, veterinarians, paraveterinarians, in-charge of diagnostic laboratories and other stake holders associated with animal husbandry in tropical countries including India.

I express my best wishes to the members of the editorial team for their sincere efforts and endeavours.

Parimal Roy

Preface

In this book we compiled the lectures delivered during the training course on "Epidemiology, Diagnosis and Control of Haemoprotozoan Parasitic Diseases" held at NIVEDI, Bengaluru during 10-19th January, 2014 for the Veterinary Officers of Department of Animal Husbandry, Livestock, Fisheries and Veterinary Services, Government of Sikkim. This book contains different aspects of haemoprotozoan parasitic diseases in animals including advanced diagnostic techniques, therapeutic and prophylactic measures, their epidemiology and control. We firmly believe that this book will be informative to the different stake holders associated with animal husbandry activities to tackle such disease more efficiently and successfully. In the other way, it will help to boost up the animal production in terms of milk yield, body weight gain and draught ability.

We wish to express our deepest sense of gratitude and indebtedness to Secretary, DARE and Director General, ICAR for their support and inspiration. Our sincere thanks are also due to Deputy Director General (Animal Science), Assistant Director General (Animal Health) of ICAR and our beloved Director, ICAR-NIVEDI, for their constant co-operation, encouragement and guidance in execution of this effort.

The financial help from Department of Animal Husbandry, Livestock, Fisheries and Veterinary Services, Government of Sikkim during the training programme is gratefully acknowledged. It is our pleasant duty to express our sincere thanks to all the external and internal faculty members for contributing their valuable lecture materials.

P.P. Sengupta
P. Krishnamoorthy
M. Nagalingam

Contents

Chapter 1

Diagnosis, Treatment and Control of Trypanosomosis in Animals

P.P. Sengupta

ICAR-National Institute of Veterinary Epidemiology and
Disease Informatics (NIVEDI), Post Box No. 6450,
Ramagondanahalli, Yelahanka, Bengaluru – 560 064, Karnataka

Trypanosoma evansi, a haemoflagellate extra cellular protozoan parasite causes a disease known as trypanosomosis ('surra'). It affects a number of species of domesticated animals in Asia, Africa and central and south America. The host species affected are bubalines, bovines, dromedarines, equines, felines, canines. Recently, it has also been reported several times from human host. The tryps are transmitted mechanically by haematophagous flies – *Tabanus* sp., *Stomoxys* sp. and *Lyperosia* sp.

Tsetse-transmitted trypanosomosis is a disease complex caused by several of these species, mainly transmitted cyclically by the genus *Glossina* (tsetse flies), but also mechanically by biting flies. Tsetse infest 10 million square kilometres and affect 37 countries, mostly in Africa, where it is known as 'nagana'. The disease infects various species of mammals but, from an economic point of view, tsetse-transmitted trypanosomosis is particularly important in cattle (also referred as tsetse-fly disease in southern Africa). It is mainly caused by *Trypanosoma congolense, T. vivax* and, to a lesser extent, *T. brucei brucei. Trypanosoma vivax* is also transmitted mechanically by biting flies, among which tabanids and stomoxes are presumed to be the most important, as exemplified by its presence in South and Central America, but also as observed in some areas of Africa free or cleared of tsetse (Ethiopia, Chad, *etc.*). Tsetse-transmitted trypanosomosis can affect camels and is a natural barrier preventing the introduction of this mammalian species into the southern Sahel region of West Africa. Horses are also highly sensitive. Very rare human cases have been observed caused by animal *Trypanosoma* species. However, tsetse transmitted trypanosomosis also affects humans, causing sleeping sickness, through infection with either *T. brucei gambiense* or *T. brucei rhodesiense*. A large range of wild and domestic animals can act as reservoirs of these humans parasites; particular care must be taken for people handling biological material that can contain infective human parasites, for example in livestock.

Chagas disease is caused due to *Trypanosoma cruzi* infection. The disease is a public health threat in most Latin American countries, although cases due to blood derivatives or blood transfusion has been reported in non-endemic regions. According to WHO the overall prevalence of human *T.cruzi* infection is estimated in 18 million cases and 100 million people are living at risk. The vectors are reduvidae bugs which are haematophagus and the most important are *Triatoma infestans* (Argentina, Chile, Brazil, Bolivia, Paraguay, Uruguay, Peru), *T. sordida* (Argentina, Bolivia, Brazil, Paraguay), *Rhodnius prolixus* (Colombia, Venezuela, Mexico, Central America), *T. dimidiata* (Ecuador, Mexico, Central America), and *Panstrogylus megistus* (northeast Brazil). The transmission by the vector is faecal contamination. *T.cruzi* infective metacyclic trypomastigotes are shed in the faeces of the bug and are inoculated into the human host by scratching infected faeces into skin abrasions usually caused by the bug in the process of feeding (blood-sucking). infective metacyclic trypomastigotes are shed in the faeces of the bug and inoculated into the vertebrate host not only by skin lesions but also through the mucosa of the mouth and, in humans, through the conjunctiva of the eyes. Trypomastigotes in the host cell transform into amastigotes, which multiply intracellularly by binary division. Trypomastigotes in the host cell transform into amastigotes, which multiply intracellularly by binary division inducing inflammatory and immunological responses *in vivo*. Amastigotes are then released into the blood stream as trypomastigotes. The latter are non dividing forms which are able to infect a wide range of new host cells but muscle and glia seem most often parasitized, or they have to be ingested by another reduvid bug in order to continue the parasite life cycle in the invertebrate host. In the *Reduvidae* bug the bloodstream derived trypomastigote forms pass along the digestive tract through irreversible morphological transformations in sequence; each developmental stage occurs in a specific portion of the insect's gut. Thus, in the stomach, most blood trypomastigotes change into epimastigotes and rounded forms (sphaeromastigotes). Epimastigotes divide actively in the vector's intestine and reach the rectum where a final differentiation results in the infective metacyclic trypomastigotes which are eliminated in the bug's faeces. The disease is manifested by pyrexia, directly associated with parasitaemia, together with a progressive anaemia, loss of condition and lassitude. Oedema, particularly of the lower parts of the body, urticarial plaques and petechial haemorrhages of the serous membranes are often observed. Abortions have been reported in buffaloes and camels and there are indications that the disease causes immunodeficiency.There is considerable variation in the pathogenicity of different strains and the susceptibility of different host species to disease. Disease may manifest as an acute or chronic condition, and in the latter case may persist for many months. Wild animals such as tigers, lions, deer and capybara can become infected. Animals subjected to stress – malnutrition, pregnancy, work – are more susceptible to disease. Like all pathogenic trypanosomes, *T. evansi* is covered by a dense protein layer consisting of a single protein called the variable surface glycoprotein. This acts as a major immunogen and elicits the formation of specific antibodies. The parasites are able to evade the consequences of these immune reactions by switching the variant surface glycoprotein, the phenomenon known as antigenic variation. The trypanosomes need severe glucose uptake from the host's blood leading to the hypoglycaemia of the host.

General symptoms in acute Chagas' disease may include fever, hepato- and splenomegaly, adenopathies and myocarditis. The acute phase usually passes unnoticed but there may be an inflamed swelling or chagoma at the site of entry of the trypanosomes. The acute phase usually passes unnoticed but there may be an inflamed swelling or chagoma at the site of entry of the trypanosomes. The chronic phase of Chagas'disease develops 10 - 20 years after infection and affects internal organs such as the heart, oesophagus and colon as well as the peripheral nervous system. The lesions of Chagas' disease are incurable and in severe cases patients may die as result of heart failure.

T. evansi: **An Emerging Zoonotic Potential Parasite**

The first case was reported from India in 26th September, 2004 from Chandrapur District of Maharashtra – a 46 year old animal husbandry man. After discovery of the first recorded case of human infection with *Trypanosoma evansi*, serologic screening of 1,806 persons from the village of origin of the patient in India was performed using the card agglutination test for trypanosomiasis and *T. evansi*. A total of 410 (22.7 per cent) people were positive by whole blood, but only 81 were confirmed positive by serum. However, no trypanosomes were detected in the blood of 60 people who were positive at a high serum dilution. The results probably indicate frequent exposure of the human population to *T. evansi* in the study area, which suggests frequent vector transmission of parasites to humans. Although *T. evansi* is not infective for humans, a follow-up of seropositive persons is required to observe the evolution of human infection with this parasite.

Diagnostic Techniques

1. Identification of the Agent

The classical direct parasitological methods for the diagnosis of trypanosomosis, namely examining blood or lymph node material, are not highly sensitive. In regions where other *Trypanozoon spp.* occur in addition to *T. evansi*, specific identification by microscopy is not possible. Specific DNA probes may enable identification of trypanosome species by nonradioactive DNA hybridization.

Direct Methods

a) Usual Field Methods

i) Wet Blood Films

Place a small drop of blood on to a clean glass slide and cover with a cover-slip to spread the blood as a monolayer of cells. Examine by light microscopy (×200) to detect any motile trypanosomes.

ii) Stained Thick Smears

Place a large drop of blood on the centre of a microscope slide and spread with a toothpick or the corner of another slide so that an area of approximately 1.0–1.25 cm in diameter is covered. Air-dry for 1 hour or longer, while protecting the slide from insects. Dehaemoglobise the smear. Fix in methanol. Stain the smear with Giemsa's Stain (one drop of commercial Giemsa + 1 ml of phosphate buffered saline [PBS, 2.4 g $Na_2HPO4.2H_2O$, 0.54 g $NaH_2PO4.2H_2O$, 0.34 g NaCl], pH 7.2), for 25 minutes.

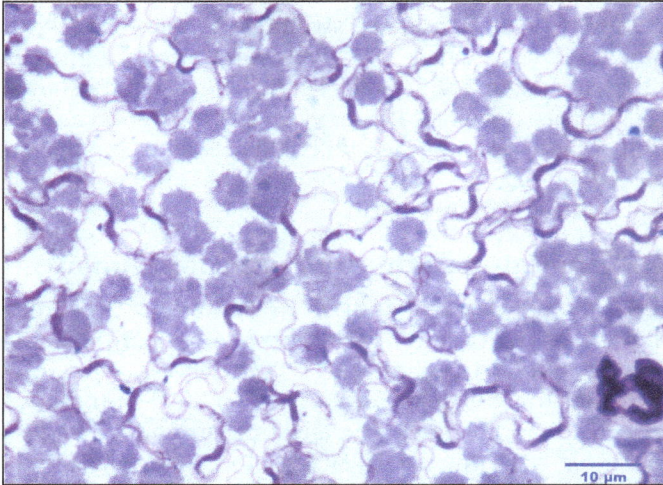

Figure 1: Blood Smear of Rat Experimentally Infected with
***Trypanosoma evansi* Showing Streaming of Trypanosomes.**

iv) Stained Thin Smears

Place a drop of blood 20 mm from one end of a clean microscope slide and draw out a thin film in the usual way. Air-dry briefly and fix in methyl alcohol for 2 minutes and allow to dry. Stain the smears in Giemsa (one drop Giemsa + 1 ml PBS, pH 7.2) for 25 minutes. Pour off, stain and wash the slide in tap water and dry.

v) Lymph Node Biopsies

Samples are usually obtained from the prescapular or precrural (subiliac) lymph nodes. Select a suitable node by palpation and cleanse the site with alcohol. Puncture the node with a suitable gauge needle, and draw lymph node material into a syringe attached to the needle. Expel lymph on to a slide, cover with a cover-slip and examine as for the fresh blood preparations. Fixed thin or thick smears can also be stored for later examination.

b) Concentration Methods

In most hosts *T. evansi* can induce mild clinical or subclinical carrier state infections with low parasitaemia in which it is difficult to demonstrate the parasites. In these circumstances, concentration methods become necessary.

i) Haematocrit Centrifugation

Collect blood (70 µl) into at least two heparinised capillary tubes (75 × 1.5 mm). Seal at the dry end by heat and centrifuge, sealed end down, at 3000 g for 10 minutes. Place the capillary tube between two pieces of glass (25 × 10 × 1.2 mm) glued to a slide. Place a cover-slip on top at the level of the buffy coat junction where the trypanosomes will be concentrated.

iii) Haemolysis Techniques

Sodium dodecyl sulphate (SDS) can be used as a reagent to haemolyse RBCs to facilitate detection of motile trypanosomes in parasitised blood samples. Both the SDS solution and the blood samples should be used at a temperature above 15°C. At lower temperatures the trypanosomes may be destroyed. Two general procedures, namely wet blood film clarification and haemolysis centrifugation, can be used.

iv) Mini-anion Exchange Centrifugation Technique

When a blood sample from animals infected with salivarian trypanosomes is passed through an appropriate anion-exchange column, the host blood cells, being more negatively charged than trypanosomes, are adsorbed onto the anion-exchanger, while the trypanosomes are eluted, retaining viability and infectivity. A simplified field method for detection of low parasitaemia has been developed. The sensitivity of this technique can be increased by approximately tenfold by the use of buffy coat preparations rather than whole blood.

c) Animal Inoculation

Laboratory animals may be used to reveal subclinical (nonpatent) infections in domesticated animals. Trypanosoma evansi has a broad spectrum of infectivity for small rodents, and so rats and mice are often used. Rodent inoculation is not 100 per cent sensitive but further improvement in its efficacy can be obtained by the use of buffy coat material. Such a procedure was able to detect as few as 1.25 T. evansi/ml blood.Inoculate heparinised blood intraperitoneally into rats (1–2 ml) or mice (0.25–0.5 ml). Inoculate a minimum of two animals. Bleed animals from the tail three times a week to detect parasitaemia. The incubation period before appearance of the parasites and their virulence depends on the strain of trypanosomes, their concentration in the inoculum, and the strain of laboratory animal used.

d) Recombinant DNA Probes

Specific DNA probes have been used to detect trypanosomes in infected blood or tissue but are not routinely applied. Although molecular methods have a potentially high analytical sensitivity there have been few convincing studies to critically evaluate the diagnostic sensitivity of these tests as compared with other techniques, such as serology.

e) Detection of Trypanosomal DNA

Detection of minute amounts of trypanosomal DNA using a PCR procedure is a possible means of identifying animals with active infections, and could have the sensitivity and specificity required. A species-specific polymerase chain reaction

(PCR) based on *T. evansi* specific antigen (RoTat 1.2 VSG) has been developed, but has not been validated in the field.

Experimental studies in buffalo showed the diagnostic sensitivity of a PCR was only 78 per cent, which is similar to mouse inoculation.

2. Serological Tests

a) Enzyme-linked Immunosorbent Assay

The principle of this technique is that specific antibodies to trypanosomes can be detected by enzyme-linked anti-immunoglobulins using solid-phase polystyrene plates coated with soluble antigen. The enzyme may be peroxidase, alkaline phosphatase or any other suitable enzyme. The enzyme conjugate binds to the antigen/antibody complex and then reacts with a suitable substrate to yield a characteristic colour change either of the substrate itself or of an added indicator (chromogen). The antigen for coating the plates is derived from the blood of a heavily parasitaemic rat.

b) Card Agglutination Tests

It is well known that certain predominant variable antigen types (VATs) are expressed in common in different strains of salivarian trypanosomes from different areas. This finding was used as a basis for a test for the diagnosis of *T. evansi*, the card agglutination test – CATT/*T.evansi* – was developed at the Laboratory of Serology, Institute of Tropical Medicine, Antwerp. The test makes use of fixed and stained trypanosomes of a defined VAT known as RoTat 1.2. Both variable and invariable surface antigens take part in the agglutination reaction.

c) Latex Agglutination Tests

A kit is available from ITM, Antwerp. It comprises a lyophilised latex suspension coated with *T. evansi* RoTat 1.2 variable antigens, PBS, positive and negative controls, test cards, plastic spatulas and a rotator. Reconstitute the antigen-coated latex particles using distilled, deionised water.

Treatment

    a) Quinapyramine salts: Sulphate (fast releasing) and chloride (slow releasing) salts of quinapyramine compound are used commonly to treat trypanosomiasis.

    b) Diaminizine compounds are also used for treatment.

For Chagas Disease

Two drugs are in common use. Nifurtrimox and Benznidazole. The latter which is now the drug of choice, is given in an oral dose of 6 mg/kg body weight for 30 or 60 days.

Fly/Bug Control

By spray of acaricides (synthetic pyrethroids, OP. CHC *etc.*).

Further Readings

1. Bajyana Songa, E and Hamsers, R. (1988). A card agglutination test (CATT) for veterinary use based on an early VAT RoTat 1–2 of *Trypanosoma evansi. Ann. Soc. Belg. Med. Trop.*, **68**, 233–240.

2. Claes *et al.* (2004). Variable surface glycoprotein RoTat 1.2 PCR as a specific diagnostic tool for the detection of *Trypanosoma evansi* infections. *Kinetoplastid Biol. Dis.*, **3**, 3.

3. Holland *et al.* (2001). A comparative evaluation of parasitological tests and a PCR for *Trypanosoma evansi* diagnosis in experimentally infected water buffaloes. *Vet. Parasitol.*, **97**, 23–33.

4. Shegokar *et al.* (2006). Human trypanosomiasis caused by *Trypanosoma evansi* in a village in India. *Am.J.Trop.Med. Hyg.* **75**: 869-870.

5. Molloy,J.B., Bowles, P.M., Jeston, P.J., Bruyeres, A.G., Bowden, J.M., Bock, R.E., Jorgensen, W.K., Blight, G.W. and Dalgliesh, R.J. (1998). Development of an ELISA for detection of antibodies to *Babesia bigemina* in cattle in Australia. *Parasitol. Res.*, **84**, 651-656.

Chapter 2

Diagnosis, Treatment and Control of Bovine Theileriosis

P.P. Sengupta

ICAR-National Institute of Veterinary Epidemiology and Disease Informatics (NIVEDI), Post Box No. 6450, Ramagondanahalli, Yelahanka, Bengaluru – 560 064, Karnataka

Theileria are obligate intracellular protozoan parasites that infect both wild and domestic Bovidae throughout the world (some species also infect small ruminants). They are transmitted by ixodid ticks, and have complex life cycles in both vertebrate and in vertebrate hosts. In India, bovine tropical theileriosis is caused by *Theileria annulata*. It also occurs in large parts of the Mediterranean coast of North Africa, extending to northern Sudan, and southern Europe. South-eastern Europe, the near and Middle East, China and Central Asia. The parasite group referred to as *T. sergenti/T. buffeli/T. orientalis* complex is now thought to consist of two species – *T. sergenti*, occurring in the Far East, and *T. buffeli/T. orientalis* (referred to as *T. buffeli*) with a global distribution. The infective stage of *T. annulata* is the sporozoite stage which is transmitted through the spp. of *Hyalomma*, a common vector tick while feeding on bovine host. Various spp. *Hyalomma* are responsible for the transmission of *T.annulata viz.,* H. anatolicum anatolicum (Eurosian countries including India and African countries), *H. dromedarii*, (Central Asia), *H.marginatum* (India, middle east), *H.detritum* (north Africa, Russian countries).

The most practical and widely used method for the control of theileriosis is the chemical control of ticks with acaricides. However, tick control practices are not always fully effective due to a number of factors including development of acaricide resistance, the high cost of acaricides, poor management of tick control, and illegal cattle movement in many countries. Vaccination using attenuated schizont-infected cell lines has been widely used for *T. annulata*, while for *T. parva* control, infection and treatment using tick-derived sporozoites and tetracycline is being implemented in a number of countries in eastern, central and southern Africa.

Chemotherapeutic agents such as parvaquone, buparvaquone and halofuginone are available to treat *T. parva* and *T. annulata* infections. Treatments with these agents do not completely eradicate theilerial infections leading to the development of carrier states in their hosts. The immune response to these parasites is complicated. Cell-mediated immunity is the most important protective response in *T. parva* and *T. annulata*. In *T. parva*, the principal protective responses are mediated through the bovine major histocompatibility complex (MHC) class I-restricted cytotoxic T lymphocytes. *Theileria annulata* schizonts inhabit macrophages and B cells. Innate and adaptive immune responses cooperate to protect cattle against *T. annulata* theileriosis. Infection of macrophages with *T. annulata* activates the release of cytokines, initiating an immune response and helping to present parasite antigen to CD4+ T cells. The CD4+ T cells produce interferon-γ(IFN-γ), which activates non-infected macrophages to synthesise tumour necrosis factor α (TNF-α) and nitric oxide (NO), which destroy schizont- and piroplasm-infected cells. B cells produce antibody that along with NO kill extracellular merozoites and intracellular piroplasms. On the other hand overproduction of cytokines, in particular TNF-α, by macrophages generates many of the clinical signs and pathological lesions that characterise *T. annulata* theileriosis and the outcome of the in fection depends upon the fine balance between protective and pathological properties of the immune system.

Diagnostic Methods

Diagnosis of acute theileriosis is based on clinical signs, knowledge of disease, and vector distribution as well as examination of Giemsa-stained blood, lymph node and tissue impression smears. *T. annulata* are diagnosed by the detection of schizonts in white blood cells or piroplasms in erythrocytes. The piroplasmic stage follows the schizont stage and, in both *T. parva* and *T. annulata*, it is usually less pathogenic and is thus often found in recovering or less acute cases.

1. Identification of the Agent

Multinucleate intralymphocytic and extracellular schizonts can be found in Giemsa-stained biopsy smears of lymph nodes, and is a characteristic diagnostic feature of acute infections *T. annulata*. Both intracellular and free-lying schizonts may be detected, the latter having been released from parasitised cells during preparation of the smears.

The schizont is the pathogenic stage of *T. annulata*. It initially causes a lymphoproliferative, and later a lymphodestructive disease. The infected animal shows enlargement of the lymph nodes, fever, a gradually increasing respiratory rate, dyspnoea and/or diarrhoe a. The most common post-mortem lesions are enlarged lymph nodes, a markedly enlarged spleen, pulmonary oedema, froth in the trachea, erosions and ulceration of the abomasum, and enteritis with necrosis of Peyer's patches. Lymphoid tissues become enlarged in the initial stages of the disease, but then atrophy if the animal survives into the chronic stages of the disease.

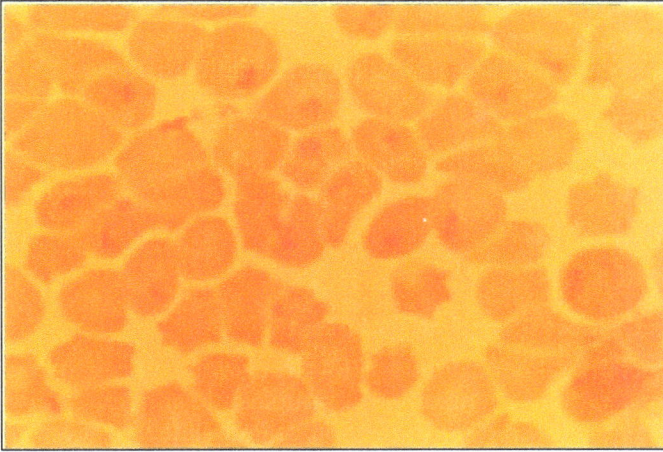

Figure 2: Blood Smear Showing *T. annulata* in the Red Blood Cells.

When examined histologically, infiltrations of immature lymphocytes are present in lung, kidney, brain, liver, spleen, and lymph nodes. Schizont-parasitised cells may be found in impression smears from all tissues: lung, spleen, kidney and lymph node smears are particularly useful for demonstrating schizonts. In longer standing cases, foci of lymphocytic infiltrations in kidneys appear as infarcts.

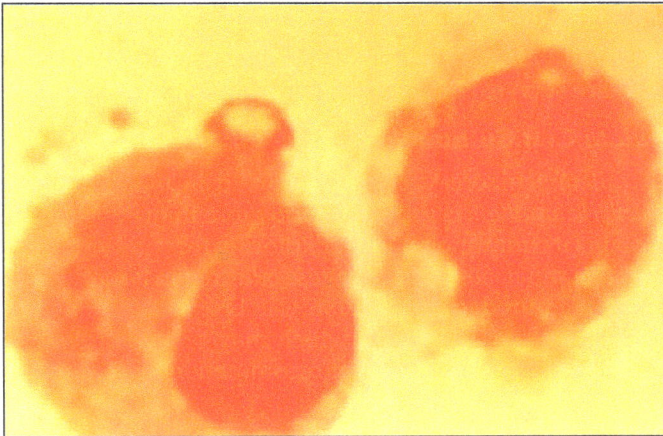

Figure 3: Schizonts of *T. annulata* in the Lymphocytes.

Both the schizont and piroplasm stages may be pathogenic. Schizonts are scarce in the peripheral blood of acutely sick animals and their presence in blood smears indicates a poor prognosis. However, schizonts can be easily detected in smears from lymph nodes, spleen and liver tissues obtained by needle biopsy of these organs. Piroplasms of most species of *Theileria* may persist for months or years in recovered animals, and may be detected intermittently in subsequent examinations. However, negative results of microscopic examination of blood films do not exclude latent infection. Relapse parasitaemia can be induced with some Theileria species by splenectomy. Piroplasms are also seen in prepared smears at post-mortem, but the parasites appear shrunken and their cytoplasm is barely visible.

2. PCR Assay

A specific PCR was developed to test whole blood samples from T. annulata-carrier cattle. Moreover, using different primers it is psssible to detect different spps. Of *Theileria*.

3. Serological Tests

i. The Indirect Fluorescent Antibody Test

The indirect fluorescent antibody (IFA) test is widely used to detect antibodies to *Theileria annulata*. Both schizont and piroplasmic antigen can be used in this purpose. Antigen is layered on the Teflon coated slide. On it antibody is given. Then antigen –antibody is traced with FITC conjugate. In this test the chance of cross reaction between different spps. of *Theileria* is minimal.

Enzyme Linked Immuno Sorbent Assay (ELISA)

Enzyme-linked immunosorbent assays (ELISA) are being used increasingly for the detection of parasite-specific antibodies. It has been successfully adapted for the detection of antibodies to *T. annulata*, and has been shown to work without cross reacting between *T. annulata* and *T. parva*. Both schizont antigen and piroplsmic antigen can be used in ELISA.

These ELISAs provide higher (over 95 per cent) sensitivity and specificity than the IFA tests and are soon expected to be available commercially.

Theileria annulata Cell Culture Vaccine

Theileria annulata schizont vaccine is utilized in many countries including India. When *Theileria annulata* is grown *in vitro* more than 300 days then it loses its virulency but retains its immunogenicity. Exploring this property such live vaccine is generated. *Theileria annulata* schizont stage is cultured in lymphoblast cell line. The produced vaccine is required to store in -196°C in LN_2. On challenge, the vaccinated animal may show a little parasitaemia which may pose a threat to non-endemic zone. Hence in non-endemic area it is not recommended.

Treatment

Buparvaquone (a quinine derivative) is a drug of choice in bovine theileriosis. It is effective against both schizontal and piroplasmic stages. This drug can be used @ 2.5mg/Kg b.wt. i/m.

Besides, some antibiotics *e.g.* oxy- and chlor- tetracycline are effective agains the schizontal stage as they cause the arrest of growth of schizonts. So they can be used only in early stages of the disease.

Vector Control

Routine spray of acaricides *e.g.* organophosphorous compound, synthetic pyrethroids are helpful in preventing ticks. Antibiotics like ivermectin can also be used routinely to reduce the load of ticks.

Further Readings

1. Urquhart, G.M., Armour, J., Duncan, J.L., Dunn, A.M. and Jennings, F.W. (1988). *Veterinary Parasitology*. ELBS.pp.1-286.

2. Bishop,R., Musoke, A., Morzaria,S., Gardner,M. and Nene,V. (2004). *Theileria*: intracellular protozoan parasites of wild and domestic ruminants transmitted by ixodid ticks. *Parasitology*, 129, S271–S283.

3. Dolan, T.T. (1989). Theileriasis: a comprehensive review. *Rev. Sci. Tech. Off. Int. Epiz.*, 8 (1), 11-36.

Chapter 3

Diagnosis, Treatment and Control of Babesiosis in Domestic Animals

P.P. Sengupta and M. Ligi

ICAR-National Institute of Veterinary Epidemiology and Disease Informatics (NIVEDI), Post Box No. 6450, Ramagondanahalli, Yelahanka, Bengaluru – 560 064, Karnataka

Babesiosis is a tick-transmitted disease caused by protozoans of the genus *Babesia*, order Piroplasmida, phylum Apicomplexa and it is characterized by haemolytic anemia and fever, with occasional hemoglobinuria and death. It is a disease with a world-wide distribution affecting many species of mammals with a major impact on cattle and man. The major impact occurs in the cattle industry where bovine babesiosis has had a huge economic effect due to loss of meat and beef production of infected animals and death. Babesiosis was first reported in 1888 by Viktor Babes in Romania who detected the presence of round, intra-erythrocytic bodies in the blood of infected cattle. Babes failed to report the presence of ticks in sick cattle but in 1893, Theobald Smith and Frederick Kilborne of the Bureau of Animal Industry of the United States, published their results of a series of experiments demonstrating that the southern cattle tick *Boophilus* (*Rhipicephalus*) *annulatus* dropping from infected cattle, were responsible for transmitting a disease called the tick fever to susceptible cattle.

Bovine Babesiosis

Of the species affecting cattle, two – *Babesia bovis* and *B. bigemina* – are widely distributed and of major importance in Africa, Asia, Australia, and Central and South America. *Babesia divergens* is economically important in some parts of Europe. Tick species are the vectors of *Babesia*. *Boophilus microplus* is the principal vector of *B. bigemina* and *B. bovis* and is widespread in the tropics and subtropics.Other important vectors include *Haemaphysalis, Rhipicephalus* and other *Boophilus* spp. *Babesia bigemina* has the widest distribution but generally, *B. bovis* is more pathogenic than *B. bigemina* or *B. divergens*. Infections are characterised by high fever, ataxia, anorexia, general circulatory shock, and sometimes also nervous signs as a result of sequestration of infected erythrocytes in cerebral capillaries. In acute cases, the maximum parasitaemia (percentage of infected erythrocytes) in circulating blood is less than 1 per cent. This is in contrast to *B. bigemina* infections, where the parasitaemia often exceeds 10 per cent and may be as high as 30 per cent. In *B. bigemina* infections, the major signs include fever, haemoglobinuria and anaemia. Intravascular sequestration of infected erythrocytes does not occur with *B. bigemina* infections. The parasitaemia and clinical appearance of *B. divergens* infections are somewhat similar to *B. bigemina* infections.

Human Babesiosis

Human babesiosis is an emerging tick-borne zoonotic disease caused by the protozoan parasites of the genus *Babesia*. Babesial infections in humans are infrequent and occur in limited geographic locations. Disease manifestations range from asymptomatic infection in healthy individuals to severe illness and death in those who are asplenic, elderly, or immunocompromised. Skrabalo was the first to identify a human infection caused by *Babesia* in 1957 in the former Yugoslavia. Earlier reports involved splenectomized patients with fulminant babesiosis. In 1969, infection with *Babesia microti* was described in a patient with an intact spleen from Nantucket Island off the coast of Massachusetts. Of the more than 70 species worldwide in the genus *Babesia,* human infections are largely due to the rodent strain *B microti* (found only in the United States) and the cattle strains *Babesia divergens* and *Babesia bovis* (found only in Europe). Sporadic cases of babesiosis due to *Babesia duncani* (isolates WA-1 and CA-5) have been reported in Washington and northern California. Genetic sequence analysis of WA-1 strain has revealed piroplasm-specific, small-subunit ribosomal DNA. Phylogenetically, WA-1 strain *Babesia* is closely related to *Babesia gibsoni,* a canine pathogen. A fatal case of babesiosis was recently described in Missouri from a strain (MO-1) that was closely related to *B divergens.* Serologic studies that test for *B microti* do not detect infections due to these other strains of *Babesia.* In a healthy individual with an intact spleen, babesiosis is rarely fatal; however, in a patient who is asplenic, babesiosis is generally quite severe and frequently fatal. In a 1998 review by White and colleagues, babesiosis was fatal in 9 of 139 (6.5 per cent) patients who were hospitalized for the disease in New York from 1982-1993. Patients with clinical illness and intact spleens are usually aged 50 years or older, suggesting that age plays a factor in the severity of the clinical response. Previously healthy individuals with babesiosis are generally older (mean >60 y) than are patients with babesiosis with antecedent medical problems (mean 48 y).

Canine Babesiosis

Babesia sp. are protozoal organisms that parasitize erythrocytes, causing anemia in the host. Many different species exist with varying host specificity. *B. canis* and

B. gibsoni are two organisms commonly known to infect dogs. Both organisms have *Ixodid* tick vectors and are found throughout Asia, Africa, Europe, the Middle East, and North America, with *B. canis* being more prevalent. Infection by *B. gibsoni* is increasing in frequency, particularly in North America, although no specific species of ticks in this region have been proven to transmit the disease. However, *Rhipicephalus sanguineus* and *Dermacentor variabilis* are believed to be potential vectors of disease. There also is evidence that some direct animal-to-animal transmission may occur, as when an infected dog with oral abrasions bites a naïve dog. Kennel settings with poor tick surveillance and control are at a higher risk for housed animals to develop babesiosis

Equine Babesiosis

Equine babesiosis is an acute, subacute, or chronic infectious hemolytic disease caused by the intraerythrocytic protozoa *Babesia equi* and *Babesia caballi*. The disease is also known as equine piroplasmosis and "biliary fever." Endemic in most tropical and subtropical regions of the world, this infection has been documented in horses, mules, donkeys, and zebras. The occurrence of equine babesiosis has been tied closely with the geographic distribution and seasonal activity of its biological vectors: species of ticks in the genus *Dermacentor, Rhipicephalus,* and *Hyalomma.* In recent times, equine babesiosis has been spreaded from its endemic tropical and subtropical zones to more temperate regions as global transport of equids has increased greatly.

Ovine/Caprine Babesiosis

Ovine and caprine babesiosis is an acute or chronic infectious disease of sheep and goats, caused by two species of *Babesia*, transmitted by ticks, and characterized by fever, anemia, hemoglobinuria and icterus.Ovine and caprine babesiosis is caused by two antigenically different species of *Babesia: B. motasi*, is a large and more virulent form, occurring singly or paired in erythrocytes; *B. ovis*, is a small form. Ovine and caprine babesiosis is widespread in tropical and subtropical regions as North Africa including Egypt, the Middle East, southeastern Europe, and South America. Ticks of the genera *Dermacentor, Rhipicephalus, Haemaphysalis,* and *Ixodes* have been incriminated as vectors. The organisms are transmitted transovarially or transstadially depending on the vector involved. Intrauterine transmission of *B. ovis* also occurs. Economic losses result from deaths among affected sheep and goats, unthriftiness of chronic cases, and the cost of control programmes. Ovine and caprine babesiosis occurs in all breeds and sexes of sheep and goats, but animals 6-12 months old have a higher incidence than animals of other age groups. The disease has a seasonal occurrence. In acute cases, affected sheep show fever, anemia, haemoglobinuria, icterus and weakness, and 30-40 per cent of affected sheep usually die. Chronically infected sheep usually are asymptomatic, except for parasitaemia and unthriftiness. Postmortem examination: reveals splenomegaly and lymphadenomegaly. Following recovery from the disease, immunity is incomplete, and most animals carry a latent infection. In cases of sudden death, the disease should be differentiated from anthrax.

Diagnostic Techniques

1. Identification of the Agent

i. Staining Blood Smear

The traditional method of identifying the agent in infected animals is by microscopic examination of thick and thin blood films stained with, for example, Giemsa. The sensitivity of this technique is such that it can detect parasitaemias as low as 1 parasite in 106 red blood cells. In blood and tissues, parasites are found most easily during acute infections. They may be difficult to detect in carriers. Treatment can also clear *Babesia* rapidly from the circulation, although the animal remains ill from their effects. Thick films can be helpful in detecting small numbers of parasites, but species identification is best in thin films. *Babesia* can be identified under oil immersion (minimum x8 eye piece and x60 objective lens) in stained blood and tissue smears. Giemsa or acridine orange is often used for staining. Immunofluorescent and immunoperoxidase labeling have also been described.

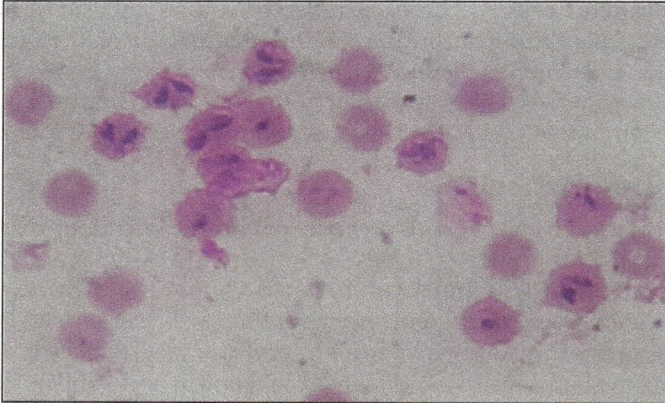

Figure 4: Blood Smear Showing the *B. bigemina* Inside the Red Blood Cells of Cattle.

These parasites are found within RBCs, and all divisional stages- ring (annular) stages, pear -shaped (pyriform) trophozoites either singly or in pairs; and filamentous or amorphous shapes– can be found simultaneously. Filamentous or amorphous forms are usually seen in animals with very high levels of parasitemia. *B. bovis* trophozoites are small (usually 1–1.5 µm x 0.5 – 1.0 µm),often paired and usually centrally located in RBCs. *B.divergens* resembles *B. bovis*, but the pairs are often found at the edge of the RBC.B. bigemina is much longer (3–3.5µm x 1–1.5 µm) and can fill the RBC. Morphological variability may make precise species identification difficult.

ii. Haemolymph Smears

As a tick-transmitted pathogen, *Babesia* parasites infect several tick tissues. Immediately after repletion with a blood meal, the tick acquires intracellular parasites, which soon escape from the erythrocytes and remain in the gut lumen for a short period of time. Sexual reproduction occurs and infective diploid cells penetrate the mid gut cells of the tick and transform to motile stages called kinetes after 72 h post-repletion. Kinetes, are motile stages of the parasite, which reach the haemolymph of the tick and infect several organs including the ovary of mated females. A good approach to identify adult females infected with *Babesia* is detecting kinete stages in the haemolymph by performing the haemolymph test. For this technique, a leg of the tick is cut with small scissors to obtain a drop of haemolymph, which is placed on a glass slide. Usually the drop is too small to be smeared so it is let dry, fixed and stained as a regular blood smear. The diagnosis is based on the observation of the kinetes, which have a vermicular shape and are usually 14.3-16.9 μ long by 2.8-3.4 μ wide, depending on the species. It is very difficult to differentiate species by the haemolymph test. Based on the biological cycle, kinetes first appear 72 h after engorgement and remain in the haemolymph until the female tick dies, with maximum kinete presence at days 5-6 post repletion. It has been suggested that *Rhipicephalus* (*Boophilus*) ticks have been adapted to start laying their eggs before kinetes reach the ovary and invade the developing embryos; the first eggs are laid at 72 h post repletion and the first infected eggs appear 92 h post repletion. By laying some of the eggs before they are infected by the parasite, female ticks ensure a percentage of their progeny to be *Babesia*-free. The haemolymph test requires an experienced microscopist since female ticks collected from cattle in endemic areas have a very low amount of kinetes.

2. *In vitro* Cultivation

In vitro culture methods have been used to demonstrate the presence of carrier infections of *Babesia* spp. has also been cloned in culture. The minimum parasitaemia detectable by this method will depend, to a large extent, on the facilities available and the skills of the operator. It is a very sensitive method for the demonstration of infection. An added benefit is that it is 100 per cent specific.

3. Animal Inoculation Test

Confirmation of infection in a suspected carrier animal can also be made by transfusing approximately 500 ml of jugular blood intravenously into a splenectomised calf known to be *Babesia*-free, and monitoring the calf for the presence of infection. This method is cumbersome and expensive, and obviously not suitable for routine diagnostic use.

4. Serological Tests

i) IFAT

The indirect fluorescent antibody (IFA) test is widely used to detect antibodies to *Babesia* spp., but the *B. bigemina* test has poor specificity. Cross-reactions with antibodies to *B. bovis* in the *B. bigemina* IFA test are a particular problem in areas where the two parasites coexist. The IFA test has the disadvantages of low sample throughput and subjectivity. The IFA test has been successfully applied to the differential diagnosis of *T. equi* and *B. caballi* infections. The recognition of a strong positive reaction is relatively simple, but any differentiation between weak positive and negative reactions requires considerable experience in interpretation.

ii) CFT

The complement fixation (CF) test has been described as a method to detect antibodies against *B. bovis* and *B. bigemina*. This test has been used to qualify animals for importation into some countries.

iii) Enzyme-linked Immunosorbent Assay

This ELISA is based on an immunodominant 58 kDa antigen identified by a number of groups in *B. bigemina* isolates from Australia, Central America and Texas, United States of America, Egypt and Kenya. A monoclonal antibody (MAb) (D6) (Tick Fever Centre, Qld, Australia) directed against this antigen has been used to develop a competitive inhibition ELISA. The antigen used in the ELISA is a 26 kDa peptide (Tick Fever Centre, Qld, Australia), encoded by a 360 bp fragment of the p58 gene, expressed in *Escherichia coli* and affinity purified. This antigen can also be used in an indirect ELISA format, but some cross-reactivity of antibodies to *B. bovis* should be expected.

In recent years a battery of recombinant antigens for the use in ELISAs has been described. Recombinant *T. equi* (EMA-1; EMA-2; Be82 and Be158) and *B. caballi* proteins (RAP-1; Bc48; Bc134) have been produced in *Escherichia coli* or in insect cells by baculovirus. Recombinant antigens produced in *E. coli* or by baculovirus have the obvious advantage of avoiding the need to infect horses for antigen production, and of eliminating the cross-reactions that have been experienced in the past with the crude ELISA antigens. They also provide a consistent source of antigen for international distribution and standardisation. Indirect ELISAs using EMA-2 and BC48 have shown high sensitivity and specificity in detecting antibodies in infected horses. Initial results from these tests are promising and further validation of the assays is underway. A competitive inhibition ELISA (C-ELISA) using EMA-1 protein and a specific monoclonal antibody (MAb) that defines this merozoite surface protein epitope, have been used in a C-ELISA for *T. equi*. This C-ELISA overcomes the problem of antigen purity, as the specificity of this assay depends only on the specificity defined by the MAb *T. equi* epitope. A 94 per cent correlation was shown between the C-ELISA and the CF test in detecting antibodies to *T. equi*.

5. Molecular Methods

Immunological methods to detect *Babesia* parasites have the disadvantage of relying on the presence of specific antibodies against those parasites, which may take days or weeks to develop in an infected animal or they are present for months after the infection has disappeared, making their usefulness very limited in acute disease cases, vaccinated animals or cleared-by-treatment animals. Molecular methods aimed to detect nucleic acids have been very useful when immunological methods do not work. Detecting nucleic acids is an indirect way of detecting the parasite so they are still considered indirect methods. However, the sensitivity and specificity of these methods are very high and over the past years many different approaches have been developed to detect *Babesia* species in their hosts and their vectors.

i. DNA Probes

Deoxyribonucleic acid probes were the first method developed to detect babesial DNA from parasitized blood. For this, DNA is isolated, purified and cloned while adding a marker, which initially was radioactive. The marked single stranded DNA is then used to hybridize to DNA present in a tissue, or a membrane. The high specificity of DNA alignment allows only the hybridization to complementary DNA, thus recognition of the desired sequence and a very specific diagnosis. Detection is carried out by autoradiography, chemiluminescence or a colorimetric substrate. *B. bovis* radioactive probe which was used by dot blot hybridization to effectively detect 100 pg of *B. bovis* DNA, estimated to be equal to DNA present in 50 microliters of 1 in 10^5 infected erythrocytes. A radioactive repetitive DNA probe, which detected 10 pg of *B. bigemina* DNA and as few as 150 infected erythrocytes. Soon non-radioactive probes were designed using chemi-luminescence or colorimetric approaches. DNA probes have also been used to detect *Babesia* parasites in tick tissues and their high sensitivity was useful for the detection of infected carriers. However, this methodology takes several days to complete, requires a specialized technician and continuous labeling of the probes; all these were disadvantages against newer methods developed afterwards.

ii. Polymerase Chain Reaction (PCR)

There are many protocols available for nested or single PCR with good sensitivity. A one-step PCR was developed for *B. bigemina* with a level of detection of 2 parasites in 10^8 erythrocytes. *B. gibsoni* was detected in 1.5 µl of blood with a parasitemia of 2 in 10^9, and *B. ovis* was detected in a blood sample with a parasitemia 1 in 10^8. Similar methodologies have been described for *B. caballi* and *B. canis* subspecies also.

iii. Reverse Line Blot Hybridization (RLB)

When multiple genera, species or strains are going to be detected in a sample of blood or tissue, this is better option than PCR. The oligonucleotides are applied with a miniblotter in an aligned format. PCR amplified products labelled with biotin, are then hybridized using the miniblotter but in an alignment perpendicular to the oligonucleotides; in this way it is ensured that all the amplified samples are exposed to each specific oligonucleotide. After a series of stringent washes, the membrane is incubated with a streptavidin-peroxidase conjugate and the signal is detected by adding a substrate using chemiluminescence. Visualization of a dot indicates the spot where the amplified PCR product recognized and bound the specific oligonucleotide. This method has been used for the detection of several species of *Babesia* including *B. bovis*, *B. bigemina*, *B. divergens*, *B. major*, *B. motasi*, and *B. caballi*, although this technique is mostly used for the combined detection of different genera and species in epidemiological studies. The most recognized advantage of RLB is that the membranes can be re-used up to 20 times, thus reducing the overall costs of the procedure. Certainly this technique is valuable when several pathogens, species or strains are present in the same sample.

iv. Real-time PCR (RT-PCR)

Real-time PCR is a technique that amplifies and quantifies a specific DNA fragment. The DNA amplified is quantified as it is being generated (in "real-time"), therefore it determines whether a specific sequence is present in the sample, and it also determines the number of copies of that sequence. RT-PCR does this by detecting a fluorescent signal emitted during the PCR reaction as an indicator of the production of the sequence being generated in each cycle; this is opposite to what happens in during the end-point PCR, where the detection of the product is at the end of the reaction. RT-PCR has many advantages over conventional PCR; it does not require post-PCR analysis because the signal is detected as it is generated, therefore, it is faster and it does not generate expenses due to electrophoretic analysis or photo-documentation. Additionally, the fact that the positive fluorescent signal is detected by the thermocycler, the sensitivity is higher compared with the in-gel analysis of ethidium bromide-stained DNA detected in a conventional PCR, and it has been reported to be at least fourfold. There are several formats for RT-PCR, the most common are based on the use of SYBR Green or TaqMan probes. RT-PCR has been reported in the infections of *B. gibsoni*, *B. microti*, *B. bovis*, *B. bigemina*, *B. caballi*, *B. canis*, and *B. orientalis*. The sensitivity of RT-PCR has been reported to be also higher than that of conventional PCR, for example, for *B. bovis* and *B. bigemina*, it was reported to detect 0.75 copies of DNA per µl of blood. Probably the only disadvantage of this methodology is the higher costs of the equipment, which usually doubles or triples the cost of a conventional PCR machine.

v. Loop Mediated Isothermal Amplification (LAMP)

LAMP is a detection method that amplifies DNA under isothermal conditions with high efficiency, specificity and speed. LAMP is based on the use of four primers specifically designed to amplify six different sequences on the same target DNA, with the aid of an isothermal DNA polymerase. By using four primers to amplify the same target sequence, the specificity of the amplification is increased, solving in part the background amplification observed in most nucleic acid amplification methods. Because LAMP produces a large amount of DNA, it can be analysed by direct observation of; a) an intercalating fluorochrome like SYBR green, ethidium bromide, *etc.*, b) the turbidity generated by magnesium pyrophosphate precipitation as a result of pyrophosphate ion by-product, or c) a newer colorimetric method using the metal ion hydroxy naphthol blue (HNB) as an indicator. This colorimetric assay is reported to be superior to the existing colorimetric assays for LAMP with regard to reducing contamination risks and expenses. Because of this, LAMP does not require of electrophoresis and image documentation post-analysis. Additionally, the isothermal conditions required for the DNA polymerase make the use of a thermocycler dispensable, reducing overall cost and time. The sensitivity of LAMP has been estimated to be of a minimum of six copies of target DNA. *Babesia* species have been detected by LAMP including *B. gibsoni*, *B. caballi*,*B. bovis*, *B. bigemina*, *Babesia canis* and *B. orientalis*. LAMP is a technique with many advantages over other nucleic acid-based detection methods and it may be advantageous in developing countries or laboratories where specialized equipment is absent.

Treatment

Control of babesiosis can be either by tick management, immunization, anti-babesia drugs or by a combination of these approaches. Chemotherapy of babesiosis is important for controling the disease either to treat field cases or to control the diseases. In endemic areas, sick animals should be treated as soon as possible with an anti-parasitic drug. The success of the treatment depends on early diagnosis and the prompt administration of effective drugs. A large number of chemical compounds have been reported to be effective against bovine *Babesia* parasites. Some of them were very specific and effective, but many have been withdrawn for several reasons. In addition, supportive therapy such as blood transfusions, anti-inflammatory drugs, tick removal, iron preparations, dextrose, vitamins (B complex), purgatives, and fluid replacements, may be necessary in severe cases of babesiosis. The first specific drug used against bovine babesiosis was trypan blue, which is a very effective compound against *B. bigemina* infections, however, it did not have any effect on *B. bovis* and it had the disadvantage of producing discoloration of animal's flesh, so it is rarely used. For many years, the babesiacides: quinuronium sulfate, amicarbalide, diminazene aceturate and imidocarb diproprionate were used against bovine babesiosis in most of Europe; however, quinuronium sulfate and amicarbilide were withdrawn because of manufacturing safety issues, and diminazene, which is widely used in the tropics as both a babesiacide and a trypanocide, was withdrawn from Europe for marketing reasons.The indiscriminate use of anti-*Babesia* prophylactic agents, including the administration of the drug at sub lethal blood levels to animals, can produce the development of drug resistant parasites, a problem that will require the development of new drugs. New drugs with a chemotherapeutic effect against babesiosis, with high specificity to the parasites and low toxicity to the hosts are desired to control the disease. Identification of novel drug targets is usually based upon metabolic pathways and cell structure. *Babesia* spp. are apicomplexan parasites that invade erythrocytes and multiply asexually with a reproductive phase, which differ from other apicomplexan that are able to invade and replicate within nucleated cells. In addition, most members of the phylum Apicomplexa harbor a semi-autonomous plastid like organelle called apicoplast, which was derived *via* secondary endosymbiotic events from eukaryotic alga. The apicoplast is essential for long term parasite viability and has been an attractive target for development of parasiticidal drug therapies.

Conventional Drugs

1. Imidocarb

It is a carbanilide derivative [3,3'-bis (2-imidazolin-2-yl)-carbanalidae with antiprotozoal activity. It is usually administered either as the dipropionate salt or the dihydrochloride salt. It is the principal babesiacide used in animals, the only one that consistently clears the host of parasites and for over 20 years, it has been used in the treatment and prophylaxis of babesiosis. The administration in cattle and sheep, is either by subcutaneous or intramuscular injection. Intravenous injection is not recommended due to its high toxicity, which may cause death in a few minutes. Imidocarb is effective at a recommended dose of 1-3 mg/kg, and it is the drug of choice for babesiosis caused by *B. bigemina, B. bovis, B. divergens* and *B. caballi, Theileria (Babesia) equi*. The mode of action of imidocarb is not fully understood, however, two mechanisms have been proposed: interference with the production or use of polyamines, or the prevention of entry of inositol into the parasitized erythrocyte, producing starvation of the protozoan parasite. Imidocarb is associated with residue problems; several studies have showed that imidocarb is retained in edible tissues of ruminants for long periods after treatment. Some authors reported high concentrations of imidocarb in the milk of ewes during the first day of treatment, reflecting its fast passage through the blood-milk barrier and a high storage due to the trapping by ionization of the basic drug in milk. A low mammary elimination of the drug is probably associated with strong binding to mammary tissue. Therefore, the use of imidocarb in food producing animals has caused some concern. Imidocarb retained in edible tissues has been related with the resistance of the drug to biotransformation processes, due to a strong binding of the drug to nuclear components, causing the formation of large deposits principally in hepatocytes, in which imidocarb is accumulated in the cell nucleus

2. Diminazene

Diminazene aceturate (4,4´(azoamino) dibenzamidine) is an aromatic diamidine, derived from Surfen (*bis*-2-methyl-4-amino-quinolyl-6-carbamide). It is marketed as a di-aceturate salt in a concentration of 45 per cent, in combination with the stabilizer antipyrine (1´2-dihydro-1´5-dimethyl-2-phenyl-3h-pyrazone-3-one), in a concentration of 55 per cent, which is added because of the short stability of the diminazene in water. Diminazene aceturate is the most used anti-trypanosomal agent and it has also been used in the treatment of bovine babesiosis. Diminazene binds irreversibly to double-stranded DNA, in the groove between complementary strands, *via* specific interaction with sites rich in adenine-thymine base pairs. The type of binding between diminazene and DNA is non-intercalative and has high affinity for kinetoplastid DNA (kDNA), which impairs kinetoplast replication and function. Moreover, diminazene inhibits the mitochondrial topoisomerase II. Diminazene aceturate is effective against *B. bigemina*, but less effective against*B. bovis* and *B. divergens*. Diminazene aceturate consists of an organic base and organic acid but once dissolved in water, it dissociates. It is usually given by intra-muscular injection at doses of 3-5 mg/kg.

Novel Anti-Babesial Drugs

1. Triclosan

Triclosan is a chlorinated aromatic compound (2´,4´,4´-tricloro-2´-hydroxyphenil ether), member of a class of synthetic 2-hydroxydiphenylethers, and exhibits broad-spectrum antimicrobial activity. It is widely used as a component of deodorant soaps, dermatologic and topical skin preparations, oral rinses, and toothpastes. Parasitic protozoa must either acquire lipids from their host or synthesize lipids *de novo* to produce the new cell membrane during cell replication. Inhibiting the ability to synthesize new membrane prevents the parasite from increasing in surface area, thereby halting cell proliferation and disease progression. The mode of action of triclosan has been associated with the inhibition of the enoyl-acyl carrier protein (ACP) reductase (FabI), a fatty acid synthase (FAS) located in the apicoplast. FabI reduces the α, β-unsaturated double bonds of the fatty acids bound to the ACP in an NADH or NADPH dependent reaction. Triclosan directly binds to FabI, increasing its affinity for the oxidized form of the co-factor NAD+, and thus locking up the enzyme in its NAD-bound form. This leaves no room for NADH binding, which is an essential step, thus bringing FAS and hence the cell growth to a halt. X-ray structural analysis of FabI bound to triclosan demonstrated that the critical binding element of triclosan is the phenol moiety. The fatty acid synthesis pathway is crucial to parasite survival as a result of a key role in membrane construction and energy reduction. In relation with *Babesia*, the inhibitory effect of triclosan on the growth of parasites has been reported in *in vitro* culture studies. The growth of *B. bovis* and *B. bigemina* were inhibited at a triclosan concentration of 100 µg/ml, while *B. caballi* and *T. equi* were susceptible to a dose as low as 50 µg/ml. In addition, triclosan prevented parasite re-growth in subsequent subcultures and all stages of the parasite appeared to be affected by the drug. No toxicity against host cells was found following the addition of triclosan.

2. Nerolidol

Nerolidol, also known as peruviol, is a sesquiterpene present in essential oils of several plants. It is a food-flavoring compound. It has shown an anti-neoplastic activity. The apicoplast of apicomplexan parasites has synthesis pathways such as fatty acid biosynthesis and isoprenoid biosynthetic pathways. The synthesis of isopentenyl diphosphate (IPP), the universal isoprenoid precursor, has long been assumed to proceed exclusively *via* the acetate/mevalonate (MVA) ubiquitous pathway, a pathway that is absent from malaria parasites. In the case of *Babesia* parasites, it has been shown *in vitro* that nerolidol can inhibit the growth of *B. bovis*, and *B. bigemina* at 10 µM and *B. ovata, and B. caballi* at 25 µM; the parasite growth is completely suppressed at 50 µM for *B. bigemina*, and at 75 µM for *B. bovis, B. ovata, and B. caballi*. The mechanism of inhibition of *Babesia* parasites is not fully unknown, nevertheless, it is known that *B. bovis* has an active isoprenoid pathway in its apicoplast. More studies with neroridol should be done to elucidate its mechanism of action, and its effect in *in vivo* experiments.

3. Artesunate

Artemisinin and its derivatives such as artesunate, artemether, arteether and dihydroartemisinin are the most common anti-malarial drugs available around the world. They are extracted from a herb called quinghao (*Artemisia annua*—sweet Annie, sweet wormwood), which has been used in the Chinese medicine as an antimalarial herb. Artemisinin is a sesquiterpene triozane lactone, contains an endoperoxide bridge essential for antibabesial activity, and has a broad specificity against developmental stages, including activity throughout the asexual blood stages and sexual gametocyte stages. Artemisinin has low solubility either in water or oil, and it can only be administered orally. Several semi-synthetic artemisinin derivatives have been developed to improve solubility in both, oil and water, for oral and parenteral routes. The major mode of action of artemisinins is by inhibiting a mammalian Ca^{2+} transporting ATPase (SERCA-sarcoplamic/endoplasmic reticulum Ca^{2+} ATPase). SERCA's role is to reduce cystolic free calcium by actively concentrating Ca^{2+} into membrane bounds vacuoles, an activity critical to cell survival. Moreover it has been showed that artemisinins targets the calcium dependent ATPases in protozoa. Artesunate has shown a growth inhibitory effect on *B. caballi*, with doses of 1.0 μg/ml, in *in vitro* cultures. However, artesunate is able to destroy *Theileria equi* but unable to destroy *B. caballi*. Artesunate inhibits the growth of *B. bovis* and *B. gibsoni*, at concentrations equal to or greater than 2.6 μM by day 3 post-treatment in a dose-dependent manner. Artesunate was also effective in the treatment of mice infected with *B. microti* at doses equal to, or greater than 10 mg/kg of body weight on days 8–10 post-infection without side effects, suggesting that artesunate could be a potential drug for *Babesia* infection.

4. Epoxomicin

Epoxomicin belongs to a family of ɑ´, β´-epoxyketone natural products. Epoxomicin was initially isolated from an *Actinomycetes* strain and it is a potent proteosome inhibitor. The proteosome, plays a key role in endogenous protein turnover. Epoxomicin inhibits its known proteolytic activities of the parasite. These inhibitory effects cause cell death by promoting the accumulation of ubiquitinated proteins within the cytoplasm. Proteasome inhibitors like epoxomicin have been proposed as anti-protozoal drugs. In the case of apicomplexan parasites, epoxomicin inhibits the growth of the organisms because it blocks the catalytically active proteasomal subunits. Epoxomicin has shown inhibitory effects on the *in vitro* growth of bovine and equine *Babesia* parasites and *in vivo* growth of *Babesia microti*. *Babesia bovis* was significantly inhibited by 10 nM epoxomicin, while a 5 nM epoxomicin treatment inhibited the growth *of Babesia bigemina, Babesia ovata, Babesia caballi, and Theileria equi*. Moreover, in the presence of 50 nM epoxomicin, the growth of *B. bigemina* and *T. equi* was completely suppressed. An epoxomicin concentration of 100 nM was needed to completely suppress the growth of *B. bovis, B. ovata,* and *B. caballi*. Furthermore, combinations of epoxomicin with diminazene aceturate potentiated its inhibitory effect in *in vitro* cell cultures. Additional studies are required to corroborate whether epoxomicin acts in *Babesia* species inhibiting the proteasome activity. An interesting observation is that epoxomicin effectively inhibits NF-κβ-mediated proinflammatory signaling and inhibits *in vivo* inflammation. Some *Babesia* species like *B bovis* or *B. canis* cause disease characterized by a systemic inflammatory response. The effect of epoxomicin on this response must also be evaluated since a babesiacidal drug with anti-inflammatory effects should be desirable for the treatment of the disease caused by these species.

5. Gossypol

Gossypol is a polyphenolic yellow pigment (1,1',6,6',7,7'-hexahydroxy-5,5'-diisopropyl-3,3'dimethyl [2,2'-binaphthalene] 8,8'-dicar-boxaldehyde), found naturally in pigment glands of the roots, leaves, stems, and seeds of the cotton plant genus *Gossypiurn*. It is a natural toxin that protects the plant from insect damage. Gossypol has been described as an inhibitor of the l-lactate dehydrogenase in protozoa. The LDH is essential for the anaerobic phase of parasite growth and it provides energy to the parasite by catalyzing the lactate from piruvate, which is the end product of glucose degradation, using nicotinamide adenine dinucleotide (NAD+) or its reduced form (NADH) as a cofactor. The l-lactate is considered as a prominent product of the transition phase from aerobic to anaerobic metabolism and it is known that in parasite LDH plays important roles in regulating glycolysis. The inhibition activity of gossypol on the growth of *in vitro Babesia bovis* cultures was 100μM. This suggests that gossypol can be an anti babesial drug, however, non-ruminant and pre-ruminant animals are particularly sensitive to the toxic effects of gossypol, and in many non-ruminant species, it causes infertility in males as well. Therefore more research should be done on the efficacy of gossypol and its derivatives against *Babesia* as well as on the effects in the vertebrate host.

6. Atovaquone

Atovaquone (1,4-hydroxynaphthoquinone) is an anti-protozoal compound. The mode of action of atovaquone against protozoa parasites is by inhibiting the rate of oxygen consumption. It inhibits cytochrome enzymes of parasites. Atovaquone seems to be very efficient against *B. divergens in vitro*. Atovaquone has been proved to be effective against *B. divergens* in gerbils (*Meriones unguiculatus*). Acute fulminating infections were effectively treated with as little as 1.0 mg/kg with increasing effectiveness up to 10 mg/kg. Atovaquone has shown to be a new drug to effectively inhibit the growth of *Babesia divergens*.

Recently, the identification of new drug targets for the control of babesiosis has been demonstrated. Inhibition of cysteine protease, reduces *in vitro* invasion of erythrocytes and the growth of *B. bovis.*

Control

a) Immunisation against Parasites

Cattle develop a durable, long-lasting immunity after a single infection with *B. bovis, B. divergens* or *B. bigemina*. This feature has been exploited in some countries to immunise cattle against babesiosis. Most of these live vaccines contain specially selected strains of *Babesia*, mainly *B. bovis* and *B. bigemina*, and are produced in government-supported production facilities as a service to the livestock industries, in particular in Australia, Argentina, South Africa, Israel and Uruguay. A killed *B. divergens* vaccine is prepared in Austria from the blood of infected calves, but little information is available on the level and duration of the conferred immunity.

The most reliable method of reducing the virulence of *B. bovis* involves rapid passage of the strain through susceptible splenectomised calves. Attenuation is not guaranteed, but usually follows after 8 to 20 calf passages. The virulence of *B. bigemina* decreases during prolonged residence of the parasite in latently infected animals. This feature has been used to obtain avirulent strains by infecting calves, splenectomising them after 3 months and then using the ensuing relapse parasites to repeat the procedure.

b) Tick Control

i. By Spray of Acaricides (synthetic pyrethroids, OP. CHC *etc.*)

Chemotheurapy by ivermectin or related antibiotics.

ii. Vaccination against Ticks

A glycoprotein (concealed antigen) of 86 kDa (Bm86), linked to the intestinal membrane, induced the production of antibodies that inhibited the intestinal cells endocytosis, without causing cellular lysis. This antigen was named Bm86, and was later synthesized using recombinant DNA technology. The use of two different vaccines, which are based on a recombinant tick antigen, showed good results in Australia and Cuba, as well as Brazil. In 1993 and 1994, these vaccines were patented in Cuba (Gavac, Heber Biotec S.A., Havana, Cuba) and Australia (TickGard, Hoechst Animal Health, Australia). The effect of these vaccines is not a direct killing of ticks, but a successive reduction in numbers, as consequence of the reduction of adult female fertility. It has been documented that tick strains have various degrees of susceptibility to BM86-based vaccines. Other proteins were isolated and tested: BMA7; Bm91; BYC - *Boophilus* Yolk pro-Cathepsin. BmTIs revealed 72.8 per cent of protection against tick larvae. Synthetic peptide (SBm7462), designed and cloned from the Bm86 with positive preliminary results. The use of chemical control associated to immunization with Bm86 is essential to achieve an efficient control of ticks. Successful immunization against the tick will permit more widespread exploitation of tick- susceptible breeds. The use of a polyvalent vaccine, with effect in different life stages, blocking important physiological functions in the tick's life allows the control efficiency to rise and makes it difficult for the selection pressure in tick population. With the discovery of new genes it is believed that a greater number of antigens with immunoprotection effect will soon be available (Cunha *et al.*, 2012).

Further Readings

1. Bock, R., Jackson, L., De Vos, A. and Jorgensen, W. (2004). Babesiosis of cattle. *Parasitology,* **129**, Suppl,S247–269.

2. Bose, R., Jorgensen, W., Dalgliesh, R.J., Friedhoff, K.T. and De Vos, A.J. (1995). Current state and future trends in the diagnosis of babesiosis. *Vet. Parasitol.,* **57**, 61–74.

3. Cunha, R.C., León,A.A.P., Leite, F.P.L., Pinto, L.S., Santos Júnior,A.G., Andreotti, R. (2012). Bovine immunoprotection against *Rhipicephalus* (*Boophilus*) *microplus* with recombinant Bm86-Campo Grande antigen. *Rev. Bras. Parasitol.,* 21(3)L 254-262.

4. Figueroa, J.V., Chieves,L.P., Johnson,G. S. and Buening, G. M. (1992). Detection of *Babesia bigemina*-infected carriers by polymerase chain reaction amplification. *J. Clin. Microbiol.,* **30**, 2576–2582.

5. Friedhoff, K.T. (1988). Transmission of *Babesia. In:* Babesiosis of Domestic Animals and Man, Ristic M., ed. CRC Press, Boca Raton, Florida, USA, 23–52.

6.   Gardiner *et al*. (1988). An Atlas of Protozoan Parasites in Animal Tissues. U. S. Department of Agriculture, Agriculture Handbook No. 651, pp. 70-71.

7.   Molloy,J.B., Bowles, P.M., Jeston, P.J., Bruyeres, A.G., Bowden, J.M., Bock, R.E., Jorgensen, W.K., Blight, G.W. and Dalgliesh, R.J. (1998). Development of an ELISA for detection of antibodies to *Babesia bigemina* in cattle in Australia. *Parasitol. Res.*, **84**, 651-656.

8.   Mosqueda,J., Olvera-Ramírez, A., Aguilar-Tipacamú,A.G., and G.J. Cantó,G.J. (2012). Current Advances in Detection and Treatment of Babesiosis. *Current Medicinal Chemistry 19*, 1504-1518.

Chapter 4

Diagnosis, Treatment and Control of Anaplasmosis and Ehrlichiosis

R. Sudha Rani

Southern Regional Disease Diagnostic Laboratory (SRDDL),
Institute of Animal Health and Veterinary Biologicals,
Hebbal, Bengaluru – 560 024, Karnataka

Anaplasmosis, also known as gall sickness, yellow bag or yellow fever, is an infectious parasitic disease of cattle caused by the microorganism anaplasma marginale. Anaplasmosis, is caused by obligate intraerythrocytic parasite of the order Rickettsiales, family Anaplasmataceae, genus *Anaplasma*. This parasite infects the red blood cells and causes severe anemia, weakness, fever, lack of appetite, depression, constipation, decreased milk production, jaundice, abortion, and sometimes death. The incubation time for the disease to develop varies from 2 weeks to over 3 months, but averages 3 to 4 weeks. Adult cattle are more susceptible to infection than calves. The disease is generally mild in calves under a year of age, rarely fatal in cattle up to 2 years of age, sometimes fatal in animals up to 3 years of age, and often fatal in older cattle. Once an animal recovers from infection, either naturally or with normal therapy, it will usually remain a carrier of the disease for life. Carriers show no sign of the disease but act as sources of infection for other susceptible cattle. Occasionally, however, some animals will spontaneously clear themselves completely of the infection and become as susceptible to the disease as they were originally. Anaplasmosis occurs in tropical and subtropical regions worldwide

Hosts

Cattle, sheep, goats, buffalo, and some wild ruminants.

Etiology

Clinical bovine anaplasmosis is usually caused by *A marginale*. An *A marginale* with an appendage has been called *A caudatum*, but it is not considered to be a separate species. Cattle are also infected with *A centrale*, which generally results in mild disease. *A ovis* may cause mild to severe disease in sheep, deer, and goats. *A phagocytophilum* has recently been reported to infect cattle; however, natural infection is rare and it does not cause clinical disease.

Transmission and Epidemiology

Some 20 tick species including *Boophilus, Dermacentor, Rhipicephalus, Ixodes, Hyalomma*, and *Ornithodoros* have been reported to transmit *Anaplasma spp. Boophilus spp* are major vectors.After feeding on an infected animal, intrastadial or trans-stadial transmission may occur. Transovarial transmission may also occur, although this is rare, even in the single-host *Boophilus spp*. A replicative cycle occurs in the infected tick. Mechanical transmission via biting dipterans occurs in some regions. Transplacental transmission has been reported and is usually associated with acute infection of the dam in the second or third trimester of gestation. Anaplasmosis may also be spread through the use of contaminated needles or dehorning or other surgical instruments.

There is a strong correlation between age of cattle and severity of disease. Calves are much more resistant to disease (although not infection) than older cattle. This resistance is not due to colostral antibody from immune dams. In endemic areas where cattle first become infected with *A marginale* early in life, losses due to anaplasmosis are minimal. After recovery from the acute phase of infection, cattle remain chronically infected carriers but are generally immune to further clinical disease. However, these chronically infected cattle may relapse to anaplasmosis when immunosuppressed (*e.g.* by corticosteroids), when infected with other pathogens, or after splenectomy. Carriers serve as a reservoir for further transmission. Serious losses occur when mature cattle with no previous exposure are moved into endemic areas or under endemically unstable situations when transmission rates are insufficient to ensure that all cattle are infected before reaching the more susceptible adult age.

Clinical Signs

In animals <1 yr old anaplasmosis is usually subclinical, in yearlings and 2 yr olds it is moderately severe, and in older cattle it is severe and often fatal. Anaplasmosis is characterized by progressive anemia due to extravascular destruction of infected and uninfected erythrocytes. The prepatent period of *A marginale* is directly related to the infective dose and typically ranges from 15–36 days (although it may be as long as 100 days). After the prepatent period, peracute (most severe but rare), acute, or chronic anaplasmosis may follow. Rickettsemia approximately doubles every 24 hr during the exponential growth phase. Generally, 10–30 per cent of erythrocytes are infected at peak rickettsemia, although this figure may be as high as 65 per cent. RBC count, PCV, and hemoglobin values are all severely reduced. Macrocytic anemia with circulating reticulocytes may be present late in the disease.

Animals with peracute infections succumb within a few hours of the onset of clinical signs. Acutely infected animals lose condition rapidly. Milk production falls. Inappetence, loss of coordination, breathlessness when exerted, and a rapid bounding pulse are usually evident in the late stages. The urine may be brown but, in contrast to babesiosis, hemoglobinuria does not occur. A transient febrile response, with the body temperature rarely exceeding 106°F (41°C) occurs at about the time of peak rickettsemia. Mucous membranes appear pale and then yellow. Pregnant cows may abort. Surviving cattle convalesce over several weeks, during which hematologic parameters gradually return to normal.*Bos indicus* breeds of cattle appear to possess a greater resistance to *A marginale* infection than *B taurus* breeds, but variation of resistance of individuals within breeds of both species occurs. Differences in virulence between *Anaplasma* strains and the level and duration of the rickettsemia also play a role in the severity of clinical manifestations.

Lesions

Lesions are typical of those found in animals with anemia due to erythrophagocytosis. The carcasses of cattle that die from anaplasmosis are generally markedly anemic and jaundiced. Blood is thin and watery. The spleen is characteristically enlarged and soft, with prominent follicles. The liver may be mottled and yellow-orange. The gallbladder is often distended and contains thick brown or green bile. Hepatic and mediastinal lymph nodes appear brown. There are serous effusions in body cavities, pulmonary edema, petechial hemorrhages in the epi- and endocardium, and often evidence of severe GI stasis. Widespread phagocytosis of erythrocytes is evident on microscopic examination of the reticuloendothelial organs. A significant proportion of erythrocytes are usually found to be parasitized after death due to acute infection.

Diagnosis

Microscopic examination of Giemsa-stained thin and thick blood films. In Giemsa-stained thin blood films, *Anaplasma spp* appear as dense, homogeneously staining blue-purple inclusions 0.3–1.0 μm in diameter. *A marginale* inclusions are usually located toward the margin of the infected erythrocyte, whereas *A centrale* inclusion bodies are located more centrally. *A caudatum*cannot be distinguished from *A marginale* using Giemsa-stained blood films. Special staining techniques are used to identify this species based on observation of characteristic appendages associated with the bacteria. *A caudatum* has been reported only in North America and could possibly be a morphologic form of *A marginale* and not a separate species. Inclusion bodies contain 1–8 initial bodies 0.3–0.4 μm in diameter, which are the individual rickettsiae.

Treatment

Tetracycline antibiotics and imidocarb are currently used for treatment. Cattle may be sterilized by treatment with these drugs and remain immune to severe anaplasmosis subsequently for at least 8 months.Prompt administration of tetracycline drugs (tetracycline, chlortetracycline, oxytetracycline, rolitetracycline, doxycycline, minocycline) in the early stages of acute disease (eg, PCV >15 per

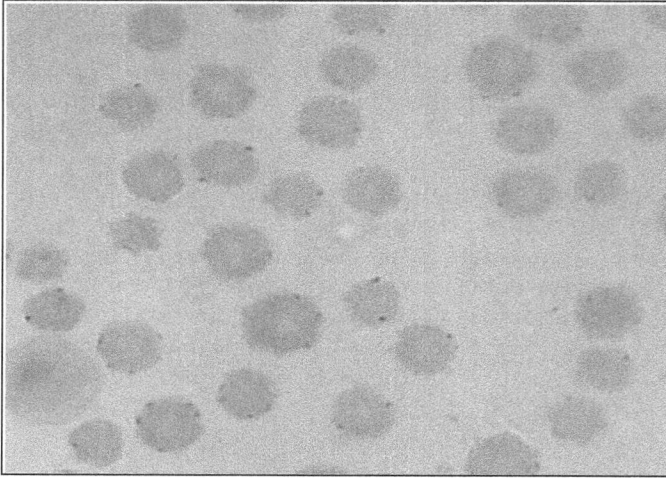

Figure 5: Blood Smear Showing the *A. marginale* in the Periphery or Margin of the Red Blood Cells.

cent) usually ensures survival. A commonly used treatment consists of a single IM injection of long-acting oxytetracycline at a dosage of 20 mg/kg. Blood transfusion to partially restore the PCV greatly improves the survival rate of more severely affected cattle. The carrier state may be eliminated by administration of a long-acting oxytetracycline preparation (20 mg/kg, IM, at least 2 injections with a 1-wk interval). Imidocarb is also highly efficacious against *A marginale* as a single injection (as the dihydrochloride salt at 1.5 mg/kg, SC, or as imidocarb dipropionate at 3 mg/kg). Elimination of the carrier state requires the use of higher repeated doses of imidocarb (*e.g.* 5 mg/kg, IM or SC, 2 injections of the dihydrochloride salt 2 wk apart). Imidocarb is a suspected carcinogen with long withholding periods and is not approved for use.

Prevention

Presently there is only one commercially available vaccine against anaplasmosis in the United States. This is a killed product that will reduce death loss, but will not prevent the disease. Two injections given 4 to 6 weeks apart with annual boosters are recommended. In rare cases, new calves born to vaccinated dams may develop an anemic crisis and die.

Ehrlichiosis

Ehrlichiosis is a tick-borne disease caused by obligate intracellular bacteria in the genera *Ehrlichia*. These organisms are widespread in nature; the reservoir hosts include numerous wild animals, as well as some domesticated species. For many years, *Ehrlichia* species have been known to cause illness in pets and livestock. The consequences of exposure vary from asymptomatic infections to severe, potentially fatal illness. Some organisms have also been recognized as human pathogens since the 1980s and 1990s.

Etiology

Ehrlichiosis caused by members of the genera *Ehrlichia.*This genera contain small, pleomorphic, Gram negative, obligate intracellular organisms, and belong to the family Anaplasmataceae, order Rickettsiales. They are classified as α-proteobacteria. A number of *Ehrlichia* species affect animals. Members of this genus of Rickettsia are found in the blood leucocytes as intracytoplasmic inclusions and characteristically produce a short febrile illness associated with leucopenia.The most important species are *E.phagocytophilia,* the cause of tick –borne fever in sheep cattle, *E.canis* causes tropical pancytopaenia in dogs.Ehrlichia phagocytophilia is transmitted by *Ixodes ricinus* and in endemic areas the prevalence of infection in young hill lambs is virtually 100 per cent.

Signs and Symptoms

Following an incubation period of seven days there is fever, dullness and inappetence which persists for around ten days.During this,although leucopenia is marked,the characteristic morula inclusions may be seen in a variable proportion of the polymorphonuclear leucocytes present. Recovery is usually uneventful, although such animals remain carriers for many months.

The veterinary significance of tick borne fever is three fold.First, although the disease in itself is transient, its occurrence in very young lambs on rough upland pastures may lead to death through inability to maintain contact with the dam. Secondly,the disease,possibly because of the associated leucopenia, predisposes lambs to louping–ill,tick pyaemia (enzootic stapylocococsis) and pasteurellosis. Finally, the occurrence of the disease in adult sheep or cattle newly introduced into an endemic area may cause abortion or temporary sterility in males, possibly as consequences of the pyrexia. In dogs the symptoms and severity of illness seen with ehrlichiosis depends on the species of *Ehrlichia* involved and the immune response of the dog. Generally, *Ehrlichia canis* appears to produce the most severe illness, and infections tend to progress through various stages.The **acute phase** occurs within the first few weeks of being infected and is rarely fatal. Recovery can occur, or the dog can enter a "subclinical phase" which can last for years, where there are no symptoms. Some dogs, but not all, eventually progress to the **chronic phase**, where very severe illness can develop. However, in practice is is difficult to distinguish these phases.Signs and symptoms of canine ehrlichiosis include fever,lethargy,loss of appetite,weight loss,abnormal bleeding (*e.g.,* nosebleeds, bleeding under skin — looks like little spots or patches of bruising),enlarged lymph nodes,enlarged spleen,pain and stiffness (due to arthritis and muscle pain),coughing,discharge from the eyes and/or nose,vomiting and diarrhea,inflammation of the eye,neurological symptoms (*e.g.,* incoordination, depression, paralysis, *etc.*). Signs of other organ involvement can appear in the chronic form, especially kidney disease.

Diagnosis of Ehrlichiosis

Blood tests typically show a decreased number of platelets -"thrombocytopenia" and sometimes decreased numbers of red blood cells -anemia and white blood cells. Changes in the protein levels in the blood may also occur. Blood smears can be examined for the presence of the *Ehrlichia* organisms. If they are present, the diagnosis can be confirmed, but they may not always show up on a smear. Blood can also be tested for antibodies to Ehrlichia, though this can sometimes produce incorrect results. Specialized testing can check for genetic material from *Ehrlichia*, and while this is the most sensitive test, it is not widely available and has some limitations as well. Generally, a combination of lab tests along with clinical signs and history are used to make a diagnosis.

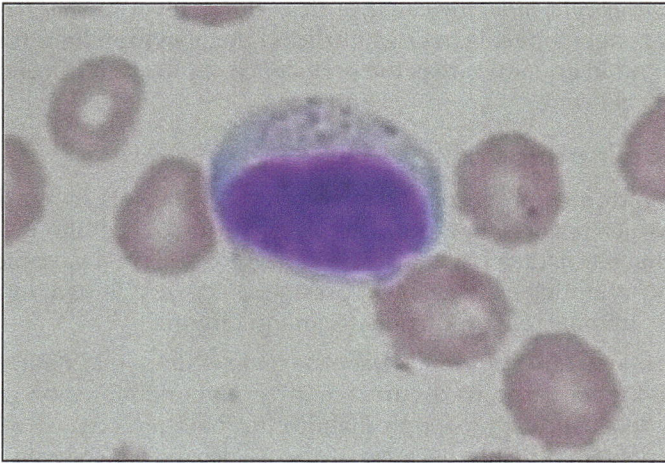

Figure 6: Blood Smear of Dog Showing the Ehrlichial Organisms Inside the Lymphocytes.

Treatment

Prophylaxis treatment depends on tick control by dipping.When tick pyaemia in lambs is a problem this measure may be supplemented by one or two prophylactic injections of long – acting oxytetracycline, each of which protects against *Ehrichia phagocytophilia* infection for 2-3 weeks. Ehrlichiosis responds well to treatment with the anitbiotic tetracyclines; doxycycline. Improvement in symptoms is usually very quick, but several weeks of treatment is usually needed to ensure a full recovery.In severe cases where blood cell counts are very low, blood transfusions may be needed.

Prevention

Preventing exposure to the ticks that carry *Ehrlichia* is the best means of preventing ehrlichiosis. Check for ticks and remove them as soon as possible (it is believed that ticks must feed for at least 24-48 hours to spread *Ehrlichia*). This is especially important in peak tick season or if your dog spends time in the woods or tall grass (consider avoiding these areas in tick season).Products that prevent ticks such as monthly parasite preventatives (*e.g.*, Frontline®, Revolution®) or tick collars (*e.g.*, Preventic®) can be used; be sure to follow your veterinarian's advice when using these products. Keep grass and brush trimmed in your yard, and in areas where ticks are a serious problem, you may also consider treating the yard and kennel area for ticks.

Further Readings

1   Veterinary Parasitology by G.M.Urquhart.Second edition.

2.   OIE *Terrestrial Manual* (2012).

Chapter 5

Role of Vectors in the Transmission of Haemoprotozoan Diseases and their Control Strategies

Placid E D'Souza

CAFT in Veterinary Parasitology, Veterinary College, KVAFSU, Hebbal, Bengaluru – 560 024, Karnataka

The importance of vectors in the fields of natural history veterinary and medical sciences and public health departments has long been realized. Vectors are assuming great economic significance since they have through the course of time become most versatile as far as their disease transmission ability is concerned. The association of insects with disease and pestilence has been recognized since the biblical plagues. It was only just over 100 years ago that a haematophagus arthropod was implicated in disease transmission. Since then, the life cycles and transmission of numerous arthropod borne infections have been studied in detail both in the field and in the laboratory. The year 1879 was a landmark one as Manson discovered the development of microfilaria in mosquitoes. In the year 1893 the discovery of the role of ticks in transmission of Texas cattle fever by Smith and Kilbourne was another major landmark in the history of arthropod-borne diseases.

The term "Arthropod" refers to invertebrate animals, externally parasitic on larger animals; many of them blood feeders in at least one stage of their life cycles. The ecological relationships between them and their hosts may be exceedingly complex, involving ectoparasites as vectors of parasites, and in some cases as reservoirs of infection as well. In their role as vectors and also as bloodsucking parasites, they have a great impact on the ecology of animal and human populations.

The term 'Vector' refers to one which spreads pathogens (Latin: vectum = to convey). A vector can transmit the disease agent either mechanically or cyclically. The major type of diseases that could have affected the early nomadic tribes must have been the arthropod-borne ones like typhus, sleeping sickness, malaria, tick-borne relapsing fever, tularaemia *etc*. A vector, according to Croll (1973) is a host which is essential for the life cycle of the pathogen, but does no more than a hypodermic needle. As an example he cited the relation between ***Trypanosoma evansi*** and the tabanid fly. James and Harwood (1969)classified vectors into mechanical carriers and obligate vectors. If an intermediate host bites or otherwise seeks out a definitive host of a pathogen it should also be considered as an obligate vector.

Feeding habits of the vector, its association with specific host species, timing of sampling, duration available for the pathogen within the vector, availability of a susceptible host for maintaining the infection chain are some of the factors controlling perpetuation of the disease. Each factor is further influenced by many subfactors needing a thorough knowledge of the parasite in question, vector species and their distribution, types of definitive hosts and their genetic makeup.

In mechanical transmission two types of vectors operate in disease transmission: 1. The first type collect the agent in their mouth parts and directly transfer it to the next host *e.g.* Blood sucking arthropods described as living needle. 2. The others are those vectors which pick up the causal agent in their legs, body hairs or proboscis as by flies and moths. They are designated as living swabs. In both the cases infection is being brought about by mere surface contact with the contaminated media.

Infectivity of a mechanical vector declines sharply with time and becomes totally inefficient within a short time. Mechanical transmission is a character of the pathogen and not of the vector. Elimination of the vector need not totally eliminate the infection but will only reduce the incidence rate. Another factor which influences the efficacy of spread of a disease here is the role of an organic medium which favours the spread of mechanical transmission.

In biological transmission, intervention of a vector seems mandatory for an efficient spread of the pathogen. The role of insects, therefore, is very important here and their control is a major weapon in disease control. Biologically transmitted pathogens undergo a cycle of development in the vector. Consequently there is a period of incubation during which the infection does not spread. When this period is over, the vector is infective and remains so for the rest of its life. Vectors transmitting pathogens by biological means are in strict sense the definitive hosts.

Broadly, five factors influence the process of dissemination and establishment of the disease.

1. **The manner in which the agent is released from the vertebrate host:** If the pathogen is restricted to blood or tissues and are to be transmitted by blood sucking or biting arthropods, the process is designated as 'active egress'. If the agent escapes from the host in feces, urine, tear *etc.* and other excretions and are transmitted by coprophagous insects, the process is called 'Passive egress'.

2. **Mode of vector infection:** This depends on the manner of egress of the agent from the host, habits of the vector, vector's innate characters. Vectors are blood sucking, tissue biting or those feeding on contaminated exudates. Attraction of vectors to certain species of hosts or to certain individuals is influenced by body odour differences, body temperature, certain chemicals emanated from the host, level of CO_2 in exhaled air, skin colour *etc*. Studies have shown that such factors greatly influenced preferential affinity of vectors to specific hosts and thereby the character of the epidemics. The mode of infection is also dependent on the barriers present in various organs of the vector, which indirectly depends on the concentration of the agent in the host and the time of feeding.

3. **Course of infection in the vector:** The agents have different predilection sites inside the vector and the cause of infection depended on (a) the time required to amplify inside the vector, (b) whether the agent actively multiplied or remained unaltered for long periods.

4 **Manner of release of the pathogen from the vector:** This is dependent on the action of the vector itself. In mosquitoes, the pathogen is automatically injected while feeding, in ticks they are expelled along with saliva while feeding, fleas disgorge plague bacilli by vomiting: bugs discard the pathogen by defecation while feeding or shortly thereafter, lice and mites which have the pathogen in their tissues contaminate the wounds created by scratching process of the host in turn resulting in crushing of the vectors. Some vectors are ingested by the host and the pathogen leaves the vector by heat or while being digested (Snail, earthworm).

5. **Combination of circumstances required for infecting the vertebrate host:** Vectors may go in search of hosts (mosquitoes, flies) or merely place themselves in vantage perches (ticks, lice, mites) such as on leaf blades, branches, shrubs and wait for a potential host to approach the site. They are activated by vibration during the passage of the host. The height of plant and the other sites selected by different stages of the vectors often determine the species of host encountered.

The transmission of pathogens by vectors is also, profoundly influenced by a number of other parameters like:

1. Vector density
2. Population density of the host
3. Environmental conditions
4. Spectrum of pathogen susceptibility of the vector
5. Geographic distribution of specific species and sub-species of the vector

Such knowledge will immensely help us in understanding vector-borne diseases and in designing strategies for their control. Vector science involves the study of vector-pathogen and vector-vertebrate interactions. Vector-pathogen association ranges from facultative relationships to highly specific obligatory relationships. In obligatory relationships, the pathogens do multiply in the vector and show a definite infective cycle. Evolution of blood feeding habit (haematophagy) is one of the greatest attributes of vectors which transmit pathogens of vertebrates including man. Many evidences especially the studies on Diptera indicate that haematophagy in insects originated at a time much before mammals were differentiated into an ecologically important group.

It is interesting and suggestive to note that even to this date many blood sucking groups among Diptera (flies) still use amphibians and reptiles as hosts. At least three major routes could be suggested for the evolution of haematophagy.

1. It could have developed as an offshoot of the scavenging and predatory habits exhibited by the progenitors of the arthropods in question which must have been inhabitants of lair or nest of the would be hosts. The blood sucking Triatomine bugs and their close relatives, the reduvid bugs illustrate the evolution of haematophagy from predatory habits. Fleas, the larvae of which are detritous feeders and adults blood sucking could be one of the examples of development of haematophagy from scavenging habit.

2. A possible second route of evolution of blood sucking habit would be chance feeding encounters perhaps initially on proteinaceous secretions carried a step further into a more purposive relationship.

3. Secondary haematophagy, a third possible route in the evolution of blood feeding habit is seen in many Diptera. *Fannia flavipalpis* and *Hydrotaea armipes* are reported to be in association with and imbibing blood made available by tabanids.

The role of vectors in the transmission of many important parasitic diseases is well established. Vector borne diseases account for more than half of the disease problems encountered in animals and seriously affects productivity and health. In spite of the predominance of vectors and vector borne parasitic infections in tropical countries including India this area of study has generally remained neglected. Research work has been largely confined to the study of incidence or superficial aspects of biology and taxonomy of vectors. It is needless to state that vector control could lead to effective eradication of serious parasitic problems such as *Theileriosis, Babesiosis, Trypanasomosis* and many other commonly encountered infections in the field. Attention with regards to the control of vectors has always focussed on the use of chemicals even though they have undesirable effects on the environment. Many a time constant use of pesticides has led to its inefficacy and there has been a serious problem of pestilence in livestock farms and in human dwellings. This has more and more prompted the consideration of alternate methods of control such as biological, genetic and other methods. There have however been great strides in the application of immunological and biotechnological methods to develop vaccines against vectors and vector borne parasites.

The vaccines developed against *Theileria annulata, Babesia bovis* and *Boophilus microplus* bear testimony to this statement. In order to combat vector borne disease either the parasites or the vector should be controlled. It is generally believed that vector control is more appropriate. The control of vectors faces two important challenges namely - the development of resistance to insecticides and pesticides and the environmental pollution caused due to the constant application of insecticides and pesticides. Therefore it is desirable to have alternate strategies, which do not involve resistance among the vectors. Genetic control or autocidal control is one such method.

The main objectives of vector control are to keep the vector density at the low level to minimise vector-reservoir contact and to curtail the longevity of vector species to interrupt disease transmission.

This approach which should be carried out prudently and skillfully is naturalisitic and involves an attempt to extend and intensity natural factors which limit vector breeding, survival and contact with man. But these measures have many constraints and limitations *viz.*

1. Selective applications,
2. Require high degree of inter-sectoral coordination,
3. Capital investment of some of the methods is high,
4. Maintenance is very essential
5. Active and sustained community involvement.

Different Approaches and Systems in the Control of Arthropod Pests and Vectors

Arthropod parasites (ectoparasites) are a major cause of production losses in livestock throughout the world. In addition, many arthropod species act as vectors of disease for both animals and humans. Treatment with various drugs to reduce or eliminate ectoparasites is therefore often required to maintain health and to prevent economic loss in food animals. The choice and use of ectoparasiticides depends to a large extent on husbandry and management practices, as well as on the type of ectoparasite causing the infestation. Accurate identification of the parasite or correct diagnosis based on clinical signs is necessary for selection of the appropriate drug. The selected agent can be administered or applied directly to the animal, or introduced into the environment to reduce the arthropod population to a level that is no longer of economic or health consequence. Parasites that live permanently on the skin, such as lice, keds, and mites, are controlled by directly treating the host. Semi-permanent parasites (ticks, flies, etc) are less easily controlled because only a small proportion of the population can be treated at any one time, and other hosts may maintain them.

Some tick and mite species stay on the host only long enough to feed, which may be as short as 30 min, or as long as 21 days. Biting flies, such as the horn fly, can be found continuously on the backs and undersides of cattle, where they suck blood up to 20 times a day; other biting flies (such as stable flies and horse flies) and mosquitos feed to repletion, then leave the animal to lay eggs. Non biting flies, such as the face fly or the house fly, may visit infrequently but can be very annoying and may transmit disease agents. Larvae of certain blowflies live on the skin or in tissues of sheep and other animals and cause cutaneous myiasis. Larvae of other flies spend several months inside animals, eg, nasal bots in the nasal passages of sheep and goats, bots in the stomach of horses, and cattle grubs or warbles in the spinal canal, back, or esophageal tissues.

Personal Protection Measures

1. Anti-Adult Measures

Several personal protection measures are available for providing protection against insect bite. They can be used as supplementary measures in remote and inaccessible areas or against exophilic and endophagic vector species depending upon their feasibility, cost effectiveness and sustainability.

- i. Physical Method This include protective clothing's, use of bed nets, screening of windows/doors *etc.*
- ii. Repellents these are chemicals that prevent insect damage to plants or animals by rendering them unattractive, unpalatable, or offensive. Thus, repellents include a wide range of chemicals, from volatile substances active in the vapour phase to protect humans against biting flies, and mosquitoes DMP (Dimethyl phthalate) and DEET (Diethyl toluamide) to persistent chemicals such as Bordeaux mixture which act as feeding deterrents to foliage feeders. Many species of ticks throughout the world are serious pests of man and animals. Current methods of protection from attack by ticks depend upon personal protection through the use of repellents.

Space Spraying by mist. Thermal Fogging or ULV Spray

Space spraying has been successfully used to control the out breaks of vector-borne diseases such as malaria, dengue, Japanese encephalitis, western equine encephalitis *etc.* The space spray is usually undertaken to control the resting population of mosquitoes either by using the natural pyrethrin extract diluted in Kerosene oil or malathion during out break situations to interrupt the disease transmission by crisis. This is done in the form of mist, chemical fogging or ULV spray.

2. Anti-larval Measures

Anti larval measures are used as an adjunct to other methods of control and are rarely used as main method of control except against container breeding species or against those mosquito species which bred in confined or specific small water bodies such as *Aedes aegypti, Anopheles stephensi* and *An. sundaicus.* Anti larval measures can also be tried in an area where vector species are resistant to commonly used insecticide or exhibit exophily and exophagy or under those situations where adulticide measures are not cost effective or tend to endanger the environment.

Antilarval measures in tropical countries are mainly used in urban or peri urban areas. These measures can be used in certain specialised situation like mining, irrigation, wells, tanks *etc.* if they are operationally feasible and cost effective. The basic idea of all anti larval measures is to prevent, reduce or eliminate the breeding places.

    i) M.L.O. (Mosqito larvicidal oil - Oiling is done in situations where breeding is temporary and permanent measures may not be cost effective. Oiling of a breeding sites kill the larvae by choking their spiracles with oil film and cutting the oxygen supply. It also deters the adult mosquitoes from egg laying.

    ii) Paris green (Copper aceto-arsenite) - It has been successfully used in malaria control programme for the control of anopheline and culicine breeding. It is applied as dust or granular formulation.

    iii) Abate (Temephos and Baytex (Fenthion) - Widely used under urban Malaria Scheme for the control of breeding of anopheline and culicines mosquitoes.

Genetic Control Mechanisms

Despite the advantage of insecticides for pest control, the use of insecticide has been ecologically unsound, leading to disadvantages such as insect pest resistance, outbreak of secondary pests, adverse effects on non target organisms, objectionable pesticide residues, and direct hazards to the user and environmental pollution caused due to the constant application of insecticide and pesticide. Therefore, it is desirable to have alternate strategies which do not involve resistance among the vectors. Genetic control or autocidal control is one such method.

The use of insects to control populations of their own kind through the transfer of damaged genetic material represents a new approach that could prove to be useful for the control of a number of major insect pests throughout the world. The principal requirement for the success of all genetic control methods is the production of sufficient numbers of healthy, competitive (though genetically different) insects and their release in the right place at the right time for them to mate successfully with wild insects. Success will depend on the knowledge of how to rear the species on a large scale, how to sterilize or otherwise genetically manipulate without affecting mating ability and competitiveness and a detailed acquaintance with the general ecology and bionomics of the insect to be controlled (Davidson, 1974).

Translocations

A chromosomal translocation involves the breakage of two non-homologous chromosomes and the reattachment of the broken parts to the wrong partners. During meiosis, in the translocation heterozygotes, the synoptic forces between homologous loci result in the formation of a cross shaped figure (Belling and Blakesies, 1924). It is the subsequent segregation pattern of this configuration which can lead to reduced fertility of translocation heterozygotes and which may be utilized for insect control naturally occurring translocations are rare but can be induced either by applying chemicals or radiations.

Genetic Sexing

In genetic control programme (s), semi-sterile males are released into natural population. since the females of the insects are potential vectors and cause biting nuisance, they should be eliminated during early development stages by genetic methods. This will also help to lower the cost of mass production of males for release purposes.

Genetic sexing mechanisms utilising conditional lethal (*e.g.* insecticide susceptible gene or temperature sensitive gene) and radiation induced Y-linked translocation and a inversion been carried out for a number of mosquito vectors. These include An. gambiae species A; the dieldrin resistant semi-dominant autosomal gene was transiocated to the Y-chromosome via radiation induced translocation (Curtis *et al.*, 1976).

Sterile Insect technique

The Sterile Insect Technique (SIT) is based on the induction of sexual sterility in males through the use of radiation or chemical sterilants and on inundating natural populations with such males (Knipling, 1955, 1959). Such techniques have been extensively used for the control of insect vectors of diseases, insect of veterinary importance and agricultural pest.

The major success has been achieved in the control of the screw worm, *Cochliomyia hominivorax* (Coquerel), a major pest to livestock in the Southern United States. In this case control was effected through the competition for mating between sterile mass-reared males and the natural population of males. At present the screw worm has been eradicated from the southeastern United States.

Cytoplasmic Incompatibility

Sterility in certain crosses between strains of *Cx. pipiens* complex was first reported by Marshall (1938). Laven (1967a) made extensive studies between certain allopatic populations of *Cx. pipiens.* Such an incompatibility which can be either uni or bi directional and which is maternally transmitted has been ascribed to the presence of a rickettsial endo symbiont, Wolbachia species in the gonads. Thus, incompatibility is due to the death of the sperm nucleus in an incompatible egg cytoplasm before karyogamy occurs. As a result no progeny are produced from such incompatible crosses.

Refractoriness to Disease Transmission

The production of genetically defined lines of vector mosquitoes refractory to the development of parasite and thus incapable of transmitting the infection is one possible method of controlling vector borne diseases. Apart from selection of malaria refractoriness by old fashion animal breeding technique, ideas have also been presented as to how refractoriness might have been contrived by genetic engineering method (WHO, 1996). These suggestions include the introduction of gene coding for a transmission blocking single chain antibody (Winger *et al.*, 1987) namely an antibody against Plasmodium gamete, zygotes or oocysts which are produced in or on the stomach of the mosquito.

Integrated Vector Control

The integrated vector control may be defined as the application of one or more than one vector control method. Simultaneously or consequently in a given area to control vector borne diseases when available options are selected on the basis of epidemiological paradigm, vector behaviour, human behaviour and environmental aspects, it become selective vector control. This approach is quite appropriate but requires effective planning, technical, competence, managerial skills and sound understanding of vector and its environment.

Community Participation

WHO Aima Ata Declaration (1973) envisaged that community participation should be considered as a crucial component of Primary Health Care (PHC). The idea of commmity participation was developed with the fond hope that it will make disease control of communicable diseases was considered advantageous to improve the quality of preventive care, reduce morbidity and mortality due to communicable diseases and encourage the participation of people. Involvement of community for the success of any vector control programme assumed still greater significance as the problem revolves mainly around man and his environment. T'he community will perceive the impact of control measures which will stimulate their active involvement in PHC socially, culturally and technically.

Consequent upon the resurgence of Kala-azar in Bihar in 1977 Plague in Maharashtra and Gujarat in 1994 and Dengue/DHF in Delhi, Haryana and Punjab during 1996, it was observed that the public health education about vector-bome diseases is poor and community participation was practically nil. It is felt that for the control of vector-borne diseases, community may be motivated to co-operate and participate for the effective implementation of vector control strategy. After motivation, the community would be able to extend their full co-operation in getting their dwelling units, cattle sheds *etc.*, sprayed with insecticide and should restrain from mud plastering the insecticide treated surface for a minimum period of two months for the retention of residual effect of insecticide. Besides, the community may be motivated to undertake bio-environmental measures like removal of garbage from in and around the houses, pigsties, cattle sheds and filling of all cracks and crevices. The shelters should be made more ventilated and lighted to prevent the breeding, resting and feeding of vector species. For the success of vector control programme, there has to be frequent interactions between the health workers and the people so that they may accept the control programme as the "People's Programme" and only this approach will be fruitful for the effective implementation of vector control strategy vis a vis control of vector-borne diseases in various parts of the country.

Chemical Control

The most common method of control of all arthropods is the use of insecticides or acaricides. The agents are classed as follows:

Organochlorides

The insecticidal properties of the best known representative of this class of insecticides, DDT was made by the Swiss Scientist Paul Muller. For this discovery, he was awarded the Nobel Prize for Medicine in 1948. DDT was introduced in the market in 1944. DDT works by opening the sodium channels in the nerve cells of the insect but this agent which was used for a long time effectively is now banned due to environmental and food contamination.

Organophosphates

The next large class developed was the organophosphates, which bind to acetyl cholinesterase and other cholinesterases. This results in disruption of nerve impulses, killing the insect or interfering with its ability to carry on normal functions. Organophosphate insecticides and chemical warfare nerve agents (such as sarin, tabun and soman) work in the same way. Organophosphates have an accumulative toxic effect to wildlife, so multiple exposures to the chemicals amplify the toxicity.

Carbamates

Carbamate insecticides have similar toxic mechanisms to organophosphates, but have a much shorter duration of action and are thus somewhat less toxic.

Pyrethroids

A pyrethroid is an organic compound similar to the natural pyrethrins produced by the flowers of pyrethrums (Chrysanthemum cinerariaefolium and C. coccineum). Pyrethroids now are the main commercially used insecticides. In the concentrations used in such products, they may also have insect repellent properties and are generally harmless to human beings in low doses but can harm sensitive individuals. They are usually broken apart by sunlight and the atmosphere in one or two days, and do not significantly affect groundwater quality. Pyrethroids are however toxic to aquatic organisms and beneficial insects. These are non persistent sodium channel modulators, and are much less acutely toxic than organophosphates and carbamates. Compounds in this group are often applied against household pests and animal pests as well.

Macrocyclic Lactones (Avermectins and Milbemycins)

Avermectins and the structurally related milbemycins, collectively referred to as macrocyclic lactones, are fermentation products of *Streptomyces avermilitis* and *Streptomyces cyanogriseus*, respectively. Avermectins differ from each other chemically in side chain substitutions on the lactone ring, while milbemycins differ from the avermectins through the absence of a sugar moiety from the lactone skeleton. A number of macrocyclic lactone compounds are available for use and include the avermectins such as abamectin, doramectin, eprinomectin, ivermectin, and selamectin, and the milbemycins, moxidectin and milbemycin oxime. These compounds are active against a wide range of nematodes and arthropods and, as such, are often referred to as endectocides.

Neonicotinoids

Neonicotinoids are synthetic analogues of the natural insecticide nicotine (with a much lower acute mammalian toxicity and greater field persistence). These chemicals are nicotinic acetylcholine receptor agonists. Broad-spectrum—systemic insecticides, they have a rapid action (minutes-hours). They are applied as sprays, drenches -often as substitutes for organophosphates and carbamates. Treated insects exhibit leg tremors, rapid wing motion, stylet withdrawal, disoriented movement, paralysis and death.

Ryanoids

Ryanoids are synthetic chemicals with the same mode of action as ryanodine, a natural insecticide extracted from *Ryania speciosa* (Flacourtiaceae). They bind to calcium channels in cardiac and skeletal muscle, blocking nervous transmission. Apparently only one such insecticide is currently registered, Rynaxypyr, in the generic name chlorantraniliprole.

Insect Growth Regulators (IGRs)

Many IGRs are labeled "reduced risk" by the Environmental Protection Agency, meaning that they target juvenile harmful insect populations while causing less detrimental effects to beneficial insects. Unlike classic insecticides, IGRs do not affect an insect's nervous system and are thus more worker-friendly within closed environments. IGRs are also more compatible with pest management systems that use biological controls. In addition, while insects can become resistant to insecticides, they are less likely to become resistant to IGRs. As an insect grows, it undergoes a process called moulting, where it grows a new exoskeleton under its old one and then sheds to allow the new one to swell to a new size and harden. IGRs prevent an insect from reaching maturity by interfering with the moulting process. This in turn curbs infestations because immature insects cannot reproduce. Because IGRs work by interfering with an insect's moulting process, they take longer to kill than traditional insecticides.

Insect growth regulator is a term coined to include insect hormone mimics and an earlier class of chemicals, the benzoylphenyl ureas, which inhibit chitin (exoskeleton) biosynthesis in insects. Diflubenzuron is a member of the latter class, used primarily to control caterpillars which are pests. The most successful insecticides in this class are the juvenoids (juvenile hormone analogues). Of these, methoprene is most widely used. It has no observable acute toxicity in rats, and is approved by WHO for use in drinking water cisterns to combat malaria. Most of its uses are to combat insects where the adult is the pest, including mosquitoes, several fly species, and fleas. Two very similar products, hydroprene and kinoprene are used for controlling species such as cockroaches and white flies. Methoprene has been registered with the EPA since 1975, and there are virtually no reports of resistance. A more recent type of IGR is the ecdysone agonist tebufenozide (MIMIC), which is used in forestry and other applications for control of caterpillars, which are far more sensitive to its hormonal effects than other insect orders.

Chitin Synthesis Inhibitors

Chitin synthesis inhibitors work by preventing the formation of chitin, a carbohydrate needed to form the insect's exoskeleton. With these inhibitors, an insect grows normally until it molts. The inhibitors prevent the new exoskeleton from forming properly, causing the insect to die. Death may be quick, or take up to several days depending on the insect. Chitin synthesis inhibitors can also kill eggs by disrupting normal embryonic development. Chitin synthesis inhibitors affect insects for longer periods of time than hormonal IGRs. These are also quicker acting but can affect predaceous insects, arthropods and even fish.

Antifeedants

Many plants have evolved substances, like polygodial, which prevent insects from eating, but do not kill them directly. The insect often remains nearby, where it dies of starvation. Since antifeedants are nontoxic, they would be ideal as insecticides in agriculture. Much agrochemical research is devoted to make them cheap enough for commercial use.

Approaches to Biological Control

Natural enemies have been utilized in the management of insect pests for centuries. However, the last 100 years has seen a dramatic increase in their use as well as our understanding of how they can better be manipulated as part of effective, safe, pest management systems. Recent efforts to reduce broad spectrum toxins added to the environment have brought biological insecticides back into vogue. An example is the development and increase in use of *Bacillus thuringiensis*, a bacterial disease of Lepidopterans and some other insects. Toxins produced by different strains of this bacterium are used as a larvicide against caterpillars, beetles, and mosquitoes. Toxins from *Saccharopolyspora spinosa* are isolated from fermentations and sold as Spinosad. Because these toxins have little effect on other organisms, they are considered more environmentally friendly than synthetic pesticides. The toxin from *B. thuringiensis* (Bt toxin) has been incorporated directly into plants through the use of genetic engineering. Other biological insecticides include products based on entomopathogenic fungi (*e.g. Beauveria bassiana, Metarhizium anisopliae*).

Role of filamentous fungi in Tick control, some of the fungi used were as follows

Metarhizium flavoviridae, Metarhizium anisopliae, Hirsutella thompsoni, Beauveria bassiana Paecilomyces fumosoroseus and Verticillium lecarii. Use of leguminous plants in tick control: *Stylosanthes scabra, Stylosanthes humilis, Stylosanthes hamata* and Aqueous and Methanolic extracts were used for the ticks such as *Rhipicephalus sanguineus, Boophilus microplus, Haemaphysalis intermedia,* (Fernandes *et al.,* 1999).

Methods of Treatment

Products are available for both parenteral administration and for topical application by various methods including dips, sprays, pour-ons, spot-ons, dusting powders, and ear tags. The method used depends on the target parasite and host. Ectoparasiticides that act systemically may be given parenterally or applied topically to the skin, where the active ingredient is absorbed percutaneously and taken up into the circulation. Many of the endectocides are now available as either SC or IM injections or as pour-on preparations acting systemically. Dusting powders have been widely used for the topical treatment of ectoparasite infestation but have been largely superseded by other methods of application. Many of the earlier organochlorine, organophosphate, and pyrethroid insecticides were formulated with an inert base, or bulking agent, for direct topical application. Accurate dosing may be difficult as the recommended dose rates are often loosely based on the size of the animal. Powders also have limited residual activity, necessitating frequent reapplication. Hand application of insecticides as washes, ointments (especially to skin or wounds to control cutaneous myiasis), dusts, spray foams, aerosols, etc, can also be done. To avoid gathering range animals for treatment, self-treatment devices, such as "back rubbers" or dust bags, may be placed in areas where cattle can rub against them.

Another widely used method is spray application of aqueous emulsions or suspensions. Cattle sheds, barns, stables, and dairies are typically sprayed or misted with insecticidal sprays. The animals may be sprayed with insecticide, both to kill and repel flies. A range of formulations is available as liquid concentrates that require dilution with water to produce an emulsion for application by spray. The use of microencapsulation techniques, in which a thin coat of chemical is applied around the active ingredients, can enhance the residual activity of sprays. Dips are used for the control of mites, ticks, lice, keds, and flies in sheep, cattle, goats, and horses. These may either be by full-body immersion or more shallow baths that cover only the legs and lower body. With immersion or plunge dipping, animals are either made to swim in straight swim-through or circular dip baths or are cage dipped for a prescribed period of time in strict accordance to manufacturer's instructions. Sheep dip formulations may deplete from the vat faster than the carrier fluid (stripping dips) to maintain therapeutic or prophylactic concentrations, the vat must be topped up with a higher than initial concentration of dip.

Impregnated devices include ear tags, tapes, bands, and collars in which a medium, usually plastic or some form of fabric is impregnated with the chemical, which is then slowly released onto the animal's coat. A residual life of several months may be expected from such devices. Ear tags on cattle, eg, can provide almost season-long control of biting and nuisance flies. Horses may be treated with such tags attached to halters or with strips attached to halters or to tails. Unfortunately, in a number of areas, horn flies have become resistant to the pyrethroid insecticides that are commonly used in insecticide-impregnated ear tags. Pour-ons and spot-ons contain the pesticide chemicals at relatively high concentration and are formulated to either penetrate the skin or act systemically or spread over the skin surface and act by contact. Pour-on treatments are usually applied along the backline of an animal or at a single spot on the shoulder blades using a specially designed applicator. They offer the obvious advantages of ease of use, speed, and accuracy of dose. Spot-on formulations offer a convenient and simple method of application of a small amount of the active ingredient to one or more sites.

Delivery Systems

Consumer convenience is an important factor in product choice, especially for flea and tick control. A bewildering array of systems has historically been available—powders, aerosols, sprays, shampoos, rinses, dips, spot-ons, mousses, oral tablets or liquids, and impregnated collars. However, the safety, efficacy, and ease of use of the newer spot-on, injectable, and oral application systems have rendered many of the older application technologies essentially obsolete. Some of the insecticides used for the treatment of various parasitic infestations are as follows:

1. Ultrasaber: Pour on insecticide for cattle containing lambdacyhalothrin with piperonyl butoxide used for the control of horn flies in beef cattle and calves.

2. Ultra Boss Pour-on Insecticide: A pour-on insecticide for cattle, sheep and horses containing 5 per cent permethrin and 5 per cent piperonyl butoxide. Against lice, horn flies, face flies, horse flies, stable flies, mosquitos, black flies and ticks

3. Taktic: An ectoparasiticide containing amitraz for the control of ticks, mange mites, lice and keds on cattle sheep, goats and pigs by spray or dip treatment.

4. Synergized Delice Pour-On Insecticide: An insecticide containing 1 per cent permethrin and 1 per cent piperonyl butoxide. Controls lice, horn flies and face flies on lactating and non-lactating dairy cattle, beef cattle and calves and aids in control of horse flies, stable flies, house flies, mosquitoes and black flies as well as others.

5. Saber Pour-On: A pour-on containing 1 per cent lambdacyhalothrin. For the control of lice and horn flies on beef cattle and calves, not for use in dairy cattle.

6. Saber Extra Insecticide Ear Tags: Insecticidal ear tags containing 10 per cent lambdacyhalothrin and 13 per cent piperonyl butoxide. For up to 5 months control of horn flies and up to 4 months control of face flies on beef and non-lactating dairy cattle and calves.

7. Dominator insecticide ear tags: Insecticide ear tags with 20 per cent pirimiphos methyl. Control of horn flies (including synthetic pyrethroid-resistant horn flies) and as an aid in the control of face flies on non-lactating dairy cattle and calves.

8. Butox 7.5 per cent Pour on: Prevention and treatment of flies, lice, keds and ticks on cattle and sheep. Contains deltamethrin in a ready to use suspension for external use. BUTOX 50 per cent EC Prevention and treatment of ticks, flies, lice and mange on cattle and sheep. Contains deltamethrin in an emulsifiable concentrate for preparation of solution for external use.

9. Boss pour-on insecticide: Pour-on insecticide containing 5 per cent permethrin. For fly control for lactating and non-lactating dairy cattle and beef cattle and calves, and ked and lice control on sheep.

10. Atroban 11 per cent Ec: An emulsifiable concentrate insecticidal spray for livestock and their premises. Contains permethrin. Controls horn flies, face flies, stable flies, house flies, horse flies, and black flies, mosquitoes, eye gnats, mange mites, ticks, lice, and sheep keds.

11. Atroban 1 per cent delice pour-on insecticide: Non-systemic pour-on insecticide for beef, lactating and non-lactating dairy cattle. Contains permethrin. Controls lice and flies on cattle and keds and lice on sheep.

12. Ivermectin: Ivermectin is also used in veterinary medicine. It is sometimes administered in combination with other medications to treat a broad spectrum of animal parasites. Some dog breeds (especially the Rough Collie, the Smooth Collie, the Shetland Sheepdog and the Australian Shepherd), though, have a high incidence of a certain mutation within the MDR1 gene; affected animals are particularly sensitive to the toxic effects of ivermectin. Kittens are also very sensitive. A 0.01 per cent ivermectin topical preparation for treating ear mites and lice in cats (Acarexx) is available. Ivermectin is sometimes used as an acaricide in reptiles, both by injection and as a diluted spray. While this works well in some cases, care must be taken, as several species of reptile are very sensitive to ivermectin. Use in turtles is particularly contraindicated.

Cultural and Biological Control

These measures can be directed against both the free-living and parasitic stages of ticks. The free-living stages of most tick species, both ixodid and argasid, have specific requirements in terms of microclimate and are restricted to particular microhabitats within the ecosystems inhabited by their hosts. Destruction of these microhabitats reduces the abundance of ticks. Control of argasid ticks such as Argas persicus and A. walkerae in poultry can be achieved by eliminating cracks in walls and perches, which provide shelter to the free-living stages.

The abundance of tick species can also be reduced by removal of alternate hosts or hosts of a particular stage of the life cycle. This approach has occasionally been advocated for the control of 3-host ixodid ticks such as Rhipicephalus appendiculatus, Amblyomma hebraeum and Ixodes rubicundus in Africa, and Hyalomma spp in southeastern Europe and Asia. Rotation of pastures or pasture spelling has been used in the control of the one host ixodid tick Boophilus microplus in Australia. The method could also be applied to other one host ticks, in which the duration of the spelling period is determined by the relatively short life span of the free-living larvae. However, it has minimal application to multihost ixodid ticks or argasid ticks because of the long survival periods of the unfed nymphs and adults. Predators, including birds, rodents, shrews, ants and spiders, play a role in some areas in reducing the numbers of free-living ticks. In the New World, fire ants (Pheidole megacephala) are noteworthy tick predators. Engorged ticks may also become parasitized by the larvae of some wasps (Hymenoptera), but these have not significantly reduced tick populations.

Zebu (*Bos indicus*) and Sanga (a *B. taurus, B. indicus* crossbreed) cattle, the indigenous breeds of Asia and Africa, usually become very resistant to ixodid ticks after initial exposure. In contrast, European (B. taurus) breeds usually remain fairly susceptible. The tick resistance of Zebu breeds and their crosses is being increasingly exploited as a means of control of the parasitic stages. The introduction of Zebu cattle to Australia has revolutionized the control of *B. microplus* on that continent.

Use of resistant cattle as a means of tick control is also becoming important in Africa and the Americas.

In Africa, infestations of ixodid ticks on livestock and wild ungulates may also be reduced by oxpeckers (*Buphagus* spp.), which are birds that feed on attached ticks.

Among biological agents, entomopathogenic fungi played a uniquely important role in the history of microbial control of insects. *Beauveria bassiana*, commonly known as white muscaridine fungus, attacks a wide range of immature and adult insects. *Metarhizium anisopliae*, a green muscaridine fungus was reported to infect 200 species of insects and arthropods. Both these entomopathogenic fungi are widely distributed and are soil inhabiting.

Evaluation of the biological control potential of these fungi for vectors of animal diseases has begun recently. *Beauveria bassiana* was used to control *Boophilus microplus, Hyalomma anatolicum larvae, Rhipicephalus bursa, Amblyomma americanum, Dermacentor variabilis*, larvae and adult of *Musca domestica*.

Metarhizium anisopliae was used as potential biocontrol agent for. Oil suspension of both fungi killed adults and larvae of ticks more rapidly than aqueous suspension. Between these fungi, M. anisopliae is considered suitable for the climatic conditions prevalent in our country

Other species of entomopathogenic fungi namely *Beauveria tenella, Aspergillus parasiticus, Cephalosporium coccorum* and *Paecilomyces fumosonoseus* are obligate pathogens of *I. ricinus* and *Dermacentor* sp. and are one of the potential factors to reduce natural populations of ticks.

Immunological Control of Ticks

Major alternatives to conventional acaricide treatments have been developed in recent years. Among the most important are various vaccines that have been commercialized for release to the agricultural community, including recombinant vaccines against midgut surface antigens, Tick GARD and GAVAC. Unfortunately, efficacy of tick control has not reached the levels that the inventors had hoped to achieve. According to data summarized by Willadsen, reduction in tick numbers was 56 per cent for cattle in an Australian study with TickGARD and 67 per cent for cattle in a Cuban study with Gavac. The best vaccine, recombinant Bm86, is reputed to reduce tick fecundity by 90 per cent. However, this is the highest efficacy currently achieved, with most other vaccines showing lower levels. Several exposed antigens have been expressed as recombinant proteins so far and evaluated for their efficacy as anti tick vaccine.

Tick Vaccine against Multiple Tick Species

A broad spectrum/universal vaccine is one that targets not only all stages of ticks but also multiple tick species and ideally, all species. Highly conserved antigens between tick species potentially possess the properties for cross resistance across all tick species and stages. Early experiments using *B. microplus* Bm86 demonstrated cross protection against *B. annulatus* and *B. decoloratus* infestations and partial protection against *Hyalomma* and *Rhipicephalus* spp. An important aspect of controlling tick infestations is a reduction of the transmission of tick borne pathogens. Therefore anti-tick vaccines should reduce the incidence of tick-borne diseases through reducing vector numbers in principle. The phenomenon of reduced transmission capacity of ticks fed on immunized animal has been observed with several works. Early experiments with Bm86 vaccines resulted in a reduction in the incidence of Babesiosis together with a reduced number of tick infestation. The transmission of tick borne encephalitis virus (TBEV) was prevented by the vaccination of the putative tick cement 64P in mice model, suggesting that 64P could be a potential candidate for transmission blocking vaccines. Because vaccines are expensive and involve considerable risk, a high level of efficacy is required to offset these negatives. Hence, there has been little industry enthusiasm for further commercialization of anti-tick vaccines. However, exciting new developments, such as the ability to disrupt the male engorgement factor or the administration of combined anti-tick and anti-pathogen agent vaccines, might change this picture. It can thus be concluded that a combination of methods would be required to combat the problem of vectors and vector borne diseases.

Chapter 6

Collection and Dispatch of Samples for Diagnosis of Haemoprotozoan Diseases in Animals

R. Sridevi

ICAR-National Institute of Veterinary Epidemiology and Disease Informatics (NIVEDI), Post Box No. 6450, Ramagondanahalli, Yelahanka, Bengaluru – 560 064, Karnataka

Haemoprotozoan such as *Trypanosoma, Theileria, Babesia, Anaplasma* cause devastating losses to the livestock industry throughout the world. However, it is known that most of blood protozoan parasites cause anemia by inducing erythrophagocytosis. Most of the haemoprotozoan parasites are arthropod borne and is of great economic importance in Asia and has always been a formidable barrier to the survival of exotic and cross bred cattle in India. Surra caused by *Trypanosoma evansi* has been reported in bovines in different states of India, *i.e.,* Andhra Pradesh, Haryana, Maharastra, West Bengal, Bihar and Punjab. Bovine theileriosis and babesiosis are also the most economically important diseases because of direct losses of production. With early diagnosis and effective treatment, the mortality rate can be reduced.

Laboratory investigation of animal disease is critically dependent on the quality and appropriateness of the specimens collected for analysis. Sampling may be from individual animals, from animal populations, or from the environment for a variety of purposes, such as disease diagnosis, disease surveillance, health certification, and monitoring of treatment and/or vaccination responses.

To provide scientifically and statistically valid results the specimens collected must be appropriate for the intended purpose, and adequate in quality, volume, and number for the proposed testing. Additionally, the animals and tissues sampled must be appropriately representative of the condition being investigated.

Specimens must be collected using appropriate biosafety and containment measures in order to prevent contamination of the environment, animal handlers, and individuals doing the sampling as well as to prevent cross-contamination of the specimens themselves. Care should additionally be taken to avoid undue stress or injury to the animal and physical danger to those handling the animal. Biological materials should be packaged to rigorously control for leakage, and then labelled with strict adherence to the applicable regulations guiding their transport.

General Considerations for Collection and Despatch of Samples from Live/Dead Animals for Diagnosis

Careful consideration must be given to the collection, containment, and storage of the specimens, including biosafety measures that must be in place to prevent contamination of the environment or exposure of other animals to potentially infectious materials. Diagnosis based on symptoms and laboratory examination of the relevant materials is essential for initiating treatment at the proper time. In general the following points should be duly considered while collecting materials for laboratory diagnosis.

All materials collected should be accompanied by full history of disease outbreak namely species affected, duration of disease, clinical signs, morbidity and mortality rates, disease suspected *etc.*The collected biological specimens should be transported on ice to the nearest laboratory as early as possible. If death is reported, Necropsy examination should be conducted at the earliest as putrified materials are unfit for laboratory examination. Detailed post-mortem report should be attached along with the samples collected during post-mortem. Specimen bottles with wide mouth should be used for collecting tissues. The specimen bottle should be sealed well so as to avoid leakage and clearly indicating the fixative/transport media used.

The reliability of the diagnostic testing is critically dependent on the specimen(s) being appropriate, of high quality, and representative of the disease process being investigated. Prior to sampling, consideration must be given to the type of specimen(s) needed including the purpose of the testing and the test technologies to be used. The volume or quantity of specimen must be sufficient to perform initial testing, to perform any subsequent confirmatory testing and to provide sufficient residual specimen for referral or archival purposes.

Specimens must be collected according to a sound knowledge of the epidemiology and pathogenesis of the disease under investigation, or the disease syndrome to be diagnosed. This will lead to the sampling of tissues or fluids most likely to contain the infectious agent or evidence of the infection. Considerations will include the tissue predilection(s) or target organ, the duration and site of infection in each tissue type and the duration and route of shedding, or the time frame in which evidence of past infection, such as an antibody response, can be detected reliably by the tests to be deployed. These considerations will also indicate the method(s) of collection to be used.

Some laboratory tests are not compatible with specific blood anticoagulants and tissue preservatives, such as heparin, formalin, dry ice (exposure of the test sample to elevated levels of CO_2), or even freezing. While it is critical to collect specimens as aseptically as possible, equal care must be taken to avoid contamination with detergents and antiseptic treatments used to clean the collection site on the animal, as these agents may interfere with the laboratory test procedures. Procedures requiring tissue culture of pathogens, as well as many molecular-based tests, can be negatively affected by chemicals or detergents commonly used in the manufacture or preparation of collection tools.

Specific considerations regarding different specimen types are as outlined below.

In selecting the anticoagulant to be used the collector must be aware of the laboratory tests, including PCR-based diagnostics, clinical chemistry which may be negatively affected by the presence of specific anticoagulants or preservatives. To be effective anticoagulants require that the collected blood be thoroughly mixed with the chosen anticoagulant during or immediately following its sampling from the animal.

Whole blood should be collected aseptically, typically by venipuncture of the live animal. Depending on the animal and sampling situation jugular, caudal, brachial, cephalic, mammary veins or the vena cava may be used. Care should be taken to collect and dispense blood samples as gently as possible to prevent damage to red blood cells, which causes haemolysis.

For detection of some viral, bacterial and blood parasite DNA or RNA or antibodies against some pathogens, small amounts of whole blood can be collected from the freshly opened body cavity by dripping it on a thick Whatman-type filter paper or by touching to organs or muscles with the filter paper. The blood spots can then be dried at room temperature and stored in plastic bags in a dry place. Adding a small silica gel pack to each plastic bag is recommended (Munson, 2000).

For serology, serum (clear fluid, yellow, in autolysed animals red-tinged) or plasma should be separated for the blood cells, divided into at least two sterile tubes and then refrigerated or frozen at -20° or -70° if possible until transport to a laboratory. Serum, plasma or blood from the heart of a carcass can be collected in vials during necropsy and left undisturbed for approximately 30 min to encourage clot formation, then centrifuged at approximately 2000 X G for 20 min. When a centrifuge is not available, serum can be obtained by letting the clot or blood cells settle. If blood is obtained from a live animal or a dead animal whose blood has not yet clotted, whole blood can be removed into a blood tube and stored with the tube inverted (rubber stopper down) until it clots; then the tube can be cautiously turned and the stopper can be removed with the blot clot attached, leaving the serum in the tube (Munson, 2000).

Trypanosoma evansi (Surra) Infection

Trypanosoma evansi causes a trypanosomosis known as 'surra'. It affects a large number of wild and domesticated animal species in Africa, Asia, and Central and South America. The principal host species varies geographically, but camels, horses, buffalos and cattle are particularly affected, although other animals, including wildlife, are also susceptible. It is an arthropod-borne disease; several species of haematophagous flies, including Tabanids and Stomoxes, are implicated in transferring infection from host to host, acting as mechanical vectors.

Clinical suspicion of surra can emerge from the field in case of fever and/or anaemia. Anaemia is a reliable indicator of trypanosome infection, but it is not in itself pathognomonic. On the other hand, animals with a mild subclinical infection can have parasitaemia without evidence of anaemia (Dargantes *et al.*, 2005). In enzootic areas, routine diagnoses can be made using parasitological techniques, while serological surveys can be carried out preferably by ELISA. CATT can be used to target individual animals for treatment with trypanocidal drugs.

Sample Collection from Live Animals

i) Blood Sampling

Trypanosoma evansi is a parasite of the blood and tissues. As for other trypanosomes, it is recommended that blood for diagnosis be obtained from peripheral ear or tail vein, even if the jugular vein is most often preferred for practical reasons. However it should be realised that less than 50 per cent of infected animals may be identified by examination of blood.

Peripheral blood is obtained by puncturing a small vein in the ear or tail. Deeper samples are taken from a larger vein by syringe. Cleanse an area of the ear margin or tip of the tail with alcohol and, when dry, puncture a vein with a suitable instrument (lancet, needle). Ensure that instruments are sterilised or use disposable instruments to avoid iatrogenic transmission of the infection by residual blood.

ii) Preparation of Wet Blood Films

Place a small drop of blood (2–3 µl) on to a clean glass slide and place over it a cover-slip to spread the blood as a monolayer of cells.

iii) Preparation of Thick Blood Smears (Unstained/Stained)

Place a large drop of blood (10 µl) on the centre of a microscope slide and spread with a toothpick or the corner of another slide so that an area of approximately 1.0–1.25 cm in diameter is covered. Air-dry for 1 hour or longer, while protecting the slide from insects. Placing the slide in a horizontal position, stain the unfixed smear with Giemsa's Stain (one drop of commercial Giemsa + 1 ml of phosphate buffered saline, pH 7.2), for 25 minutes. After washing and drying, examine the smears by light microscopy at a magnification of 500× with oil immersion.

iv) Preparation of Stained Thin Blood Smears

Place a small drop of blood (3–5 µl) at one end of a clean microscope slide and draw out a thin film in the usual way. Air-dry briefly and fix in methyl alcohol for 1 minute and allow to dry. Stain the smears in Giemsa (one drop Giemsa + 1 ml PBS, pH 7.2) for 25 minutes. Pour off stain and wash the slide in tap water and dry.

v) Lymph Node Biopsies or Oedema Fluid

Samples are usually obtained from the prescapular or precrural (subiliac) lymph nodes. Select a suitable node by palpation and cleanse the site with alcohol. Puncture the node with a suitable gauge needle, and draw lymph node material into a syringe attached to the needle. Expel lymph on to a slide, cover with a cover-slip and examine as for the fresh blood preparations. Fixed thin or thick smears can also be stored for later examination. Similar examination can be done by collection of oedema fluid. *Trypanosoma evansi* has a broad spectrum of infectivity for small rodents, and so rats and mice are often used.

Trypanosomosis : Similar to Surra

Bovine Babesiosis

Babesiosis is a tick-borne disease of cattle caused by the protozoan parasites Babesia bovis, B. bigemina, B. divergens and others. Babesia bovis and Babesia bigemina – are widely distributed and of major importance in Africa, Asia, Australia, and Central and South America. Babesia divergens is economically important in some parts of Europe. Rhipicephalus (Boophilus) spp., the principal vectors of B. bovis and B. bigemina, are widespread in tropical and subtropical countries.

The traditional method of identifying the agent in infected animals is by microscopic examination of thick and thin blood films stained with Giemsa.

Sample Collection from Live Animals

Samples from live animals should preferably be films made from fresh blood taken from capillaries, such as those in the tip of the ear or tip of the tail, as *B. bovis* is more common in capillary blood. *Babesia bigemina* and *B. divergens* parasites are uniformly distributed through the vasculature. If it is not possible to make fresh films from capillary blood, sterile jugular blood should be collected into an anticoagulant such as lithium heparin or ethylene diamine tetra-acetic acid (EDTA).The sample should be kept cool, preferably at 5°C, until delivery to the laboratory.

Preparation of Blood Smears

(i) Thin blood films are air-dried, fixed in absolute methanol for 10–60 seconds and then stained with 10 per cent Giemsa for 15–30 minutes. It is preferable to stain blood films as soon as possible after preparation to ensure proper stain definition.

(ii) Thick films are made by placing a small droplet of blood (approximately 50 µl) on to a clean glass slide and spreading this over a small area using a circular motion with the corner of another slide.This droplet is not fixed in methanol, but simply air-dried, heat-fixed at 80°C for 5 minutes, and stained in 10 per cent Giemsa. This is a more sensitive technique for the detection of *Babesia* spp.For serological tests: Blood with anticoagulant (sodium citrate or EDTA), blood without anticoagulant for serum.

Sample Collection from Dead Animals

Samples from dead animals should consist of thin blood films, as well as smears from cerebral cortex, kidney (freshly dead), spleen (when decomposition is evident), heart muscle, lung, and liver (Bock *et al.*, 2006; de Vos *et al.*, 2004).Organ smears are made by pressing a clean slide on to a freshly cut surface of the organ or by crushing a small sample of the tissue (particularly cerebral cortex) between two clean microscope slides drawn lengthwise to leave a film of tissue on each slide. The smear is then air-dried (assisted by gentle warming in humid climates), fixed for 10–60 seconds in absolute methanol, and stained for 15–30 minutes in 10 per cent Giemsa. This method is especially suitable for the diagnosis of *B. bovis* infections using smears of cerebral cortex.

Theileriosis

Theileriae are obligate intracellular protozoan parasites that infect both wild and domestic Bovidae. They are transmitted by ixodid ticks, and have complex life cycles in both vertebrate and invertebrate hosts.The two most pathogenic and economically important are *T. parva* and *T. Annulata.*

Diagnosis of acute theileriosis is based on clinical signs, knowledge of disease, and vector distribution as well as examination of Giemsa-stained blood, lymph node and tissue impression smears. The infected animal shows enlargement of the lymph nodes, fever, a gradually increasing respiratory rate, dyspnoea and/ or diarrhoea.Samples from live animals: Giemsa-stained biopsy smears of lymph nodes, and is a characteristic diagnostic feature of acute infections with *T. parva* and *T. annulata.*Samples from dead animals: Schizont-parasitised cells may be found in impression smears from all tissues: lung, spleen, kidney and lymph node smears are particularly useful for demonstrating schizonts. However, schizonts can be easily detected in smears from lymph nodes, spleen and liver tissues obtained by needle biopsy of these organs.

Equine Piroplasmosis

Equine piroplasmosis is a tick-borne protozoal disease of horses, mules, donkeys and zebra. The aetiological agents are blood parasites named Theileria equi and Babesia caballi. The parasites are found inside the red blood cells of the infected animals. Infected horses may be identified by demonstrating the parasites in stained blood, optimally collected from superficil skin capillaries, or organ smears during the acute phase of the disease. Romanovsky-type staining methods, such as the Giemsa method, usually give the best results. Thick blood smear technique to detect very low parasitaemia. Thick films are made by placing a small drop (approximately 50 µl) of blood on to a clean glass slide which is then air-dried, heat fixed at 80°C for 5 minutes, and stained in 5 per cent Giemsa for 20–30 minutes. For Serological tests, serum separated as described earlier and sent. For detection by molecular techniques, whole blood has to be sent in ice with proper care.

Anaplasmosis

Samples from live cattle should include thin blood smears and blood collected into an anticoagulant. Air-dried thin blood smears will keep satisfactorily at room temperature for at least 1 week. The blood sample in anticoagulant should be held and transferred at 4°C, unless it can reach the laboratory within a few hours for preparing fresh smears. In addition, a low packed cell volume and/or erythrocyte count can help to substantiate the involvement of *A. marginale* when only small numbers of the parasites are detected in smears, such as may occur in the recovery stage of the disease.In contrast to *Babesia bovis, A. marginale* does not accumulate in capillaries, so blood drawn from the jugular or other large vessel is satisfactory. Because of the rather indistinctive morphology of *Anaplasma,* it is essential that smears be well prepared and free from foreign matter, as specks of debris can confuse diagnosis.

Samples from dead animals should include air-dried thin smears from the liver, kidney, heart and lungs and from a peripheral blood vessel. The latter is particularly recommended should there be a significant delay before post-mortem examination because, under these circumstances, bacterial contamination of organ smears often makes identification of *Anaplasma* equivocal. Blood from organs, rather than organ tissues *per se*, is required for smear preparation, as the aim is to be able to examine microscopically intact erythrocytes for the presence of *Anaplasma.* Organ-derived blood smears will store satisfactorily at room temperature for several days. Both blood and organ smears can be stained in 10 per cent Giemsa stain.

Further Readings

1. Bock R.E., De Vos A.J. and Molloy J.B. (2006). Tick-borne diseases. *In:* Australian New Zealand Standard Diagnostic Procedures, Faragher J.T., ed. Subcommittee on Animal Health Laboratory Standards http://www.scahls.org.au/__data/assets/pdf_file/0008/1280852/tick_borne_diseases.

2. Dargantes A.P., Reid S.A. and Copeman D.B. (2005). Experimental *Trypanosoma evansi* infection in the goat. Clinical signs and pathology. *J. Comp. Pathol.,* 133, 261–266.

3. De Vos A.J., De Waal D.T. and Jackson L.A. (2004). Bovine babesiosis. *In:* Infectious Diseases of Livestock, Vol. 1,Coetzer J.A.W. and Tustin R.C., eds., Oxford University Press, Capetown, South Africa, 406–424.

4. Munson, L. (2000). Necropsy procedures for wild animals. With input from: W. B. Karesh, M. F. McEntee, L. J. Lowenstine, M. E. Roelke-Parker, E. Williams and M. H. Woodford; Illustrations by D. Haines). Pp. 203-224 in: Conservation research in the African rain forests: a technical handbook. White, Lee; Edwards, Anne (eds.), Wildlife Conservation Society, New York. ISBN: 0-9632064-4-3 (english), ISBN: 0-9632064-5-1 (french). Also in: http://www.vetmed.ucdavis.edu/whc/Necropsy/TOC.html, the University of California - Davis Veterinary Medical Teaching Hospital's home

page, seen: 17.06.02; also available in Porteguese, French, and Spanish from the Wildlife Conservation Society, see http://wcs.org/

5. OIE Manual of Diagnostic Tests and Vaccines for Terrestrial Animals.2012.7[th] Edition Pages 1-12.

Chapter 7

Pathological Changes in Haemoprotozoan Diseases of Animals

P. Krishnamoorthy

ICAR-National Institute of Veterinary Epidemiology and
Disease Informatics (NIVEDI), Post Box No. 6450,
Ramagondanahalli, Yelahanka, Bengaluru – 560 064, Karnataka

Haemoprotozoan diseases cause devastating losses to the livestock industry throughout the world. However, it is known that most of blood protozoan parasites cause anaemia by inducing erythrophagocytosis. Most of the haemoprotozoan parasites are tick borne and is of great economic importance in Asia and has always been a formidable barrier to the survival of exotic and cross bred cattle in India. Many animals die and undergo a long period of convalescence entailing loss of meat and milk production. With early diagnosis and effective treatment, the mortality rate can be reduced.

Trypanasomiasis

It has a wide range of hosts and is pathogenic to most of the domestic and laboratory animals. The parasite utilizes glucose and oxygen for its growth and multiplication resulting in depletion of these metabolites leading to degenerative changes in the host. Further changes develop in the organs either due to cellular damage caused by toxicants released by the parasite or due to immunological reactions. In an experimental study conducted in Rats showed lesions in liver, kidney, spleen and trypanasomes attached to the heart endocardium on histological examinations. The decrease in serum glucose and increase in creatinine level was observed on serum biochemistry.

Haematology

Progressive anaemia, number of erythrocytes and haemoglobin content are reduced to 24 per cent. Anaemia may not only be due to a failure in production due to inhibition, but also to increased erythrophagocytosis and enlarged mononuclear phagocytic systems associated with auto immune processes.

Hypoglycemia develops because the parasites consumes large amount of glucose and the liver is unable to lay down glycogen reserve. Blood lactic acid is increased, blood potassium is decreased but the globulin fraction is increased.

Lesions

Emaciated animal markedly, spleen and lymph glands are enlarged and show hyperplasia of follicles. There may be multiplication of the macrophages in sinuses and infiltration by lymphocytes and plasma cells. Later organization occurs with suppression of glandular function. Congestion of bone marrow and of the gastrointestinal mucosa may be present. Subcutis shows gelatinous infiltration with petechiae on serous mucous membranes. Serous exudate into pericardial cavity and peritoneum is seen. Ulceration of tongue and gastric mucosa is met with.

In an experimental study with different isolate of *T. evansi* indicated hyperplasia of hepatocytes and also vacuolar degeneration in liver. The testis of rats showed intersititial edema in between the seminiferous tubules indicating the damage and testicular degeneration due to the *T. evansi*. Further, the heart chamber also showed the presence of trypanosomes attaching to the muscle wall.

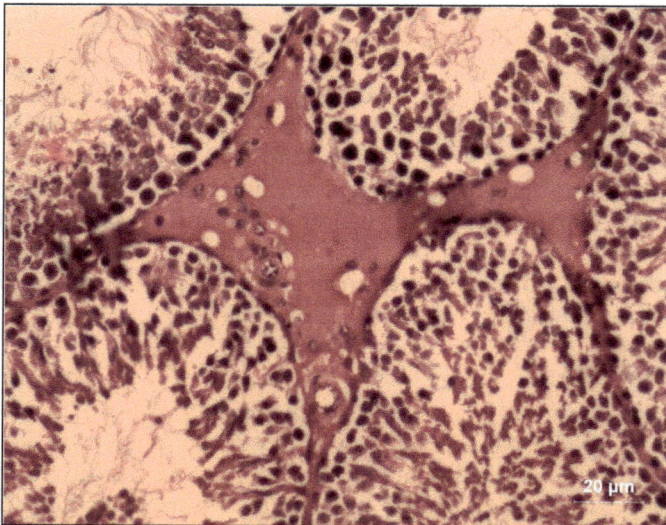

Figure 7: Rat Testis Showing the Interstitial Edema between the Seminiferous Tubules and with Testicular Degeneration.

Death in Trypansomiasis may be attributable to:

1. Endotoxin that may be released by the lysis of parasites

2. Asphyxia due to increased blood lactic acid

3. Hypoglycemia

4. Toxaemia that develops due to dysfunction of liver and the cause of hepatic dysfunction is destruction of large quantities of glucose.

5. Erythrocyte production is inhibited by toxins

6. Trypanosomes may liberate proteolytic ferments, which digesting proteins may liberate toxic products.

Theileriosis

Theileriosis are a group of tickborne diseases caused by *Theileria spp*. A large number of *Theileria* spp. are found in domestic and wild animals in tick-infested areas of the Old World. The most important species affecting cattle are *T. parva* and *T. annulata*, which cause widespread death in tropical and subtropical areas of the Old World. *T. lestoquardi*, *T. lowenshuni* and *T. uilenbergi* are important causes of mortality in sheep.

An occult phase of 5–10 days follows before infected lymphocytes can be detected in Giemsa-stained smears of cells aspirated from the local draining lymph node. Subsequently, the number of parasitized cells increases rapidly throughout the lymphoid system and from about day 14 onward, cells undergoing merogony are observed. This is associated with widespread lymphocytolysis, marked lymphoid depletion and leukopenia. Piroplasms in RBC infected by the resultant merozoites assume various forms, but typically they are small and rod-shaped or oval.

Clinical signs vary according to the level of challenge and range from inapparent or mild to severe and fatal. Typically, fever occurs 7–10 days after parasites are introduced by feeding ticks, continues throughout the course of infection and may be >107°F (42°C). Lymph node swelling becomes pronounced and generalized. Lymphoblasts in Giemsa-stained lymph node biopsy smears contain multinuclear schizonts. Anorexia develops and the animal rapidly loses condition; lacrimation and nasal discharge may occur. Terminally, dyspnea is common. Just before death, a sharp fall in body temperature is usual, and pulmonary exudate pours from the nostrils. Death usually occurs 18–24 days after infection. The most striking postmortem lesions are lymph node enlargement and massive pulmonary edema and hyperemia. Haemorrhages are common on the serosal and mucosal surfaces of many organs, sometimes together with obvious areas of necrosis in the lymph nodes and thymus. Anemia is not a major diagnostic sign (as it is in babesiosis) because there is minimal division of the parasites in RBC and thus no massive destruction of them. Animals that recover are immune to subsequent challenge with the same strains but may be susceptible to some heterologous strains. Most recovered or immunized animals remain carriers of the infection.

Symptoms observed were enlargement of local lymph gland, fever, haemorrhages on visible mucous membranes and sometimes on skin, anaemia and jaundice particularly in subacute and chronic forms of the disease. The parasite "schizont" was first detected in the swollen local lymph gland draining the site of attachment of ticks, then in other lymph glands which concurred with the onset of fever.

Main post-mortem findings were oedema and enlargement of, and haemorrhages in lymph glands and spleen, haemorrhages in subcutis and on most of the serous and mucous membranes on endocardium, pericardium and epicardium, and ulcers in abomasum which rarely extended to intestine, oesophagus, tongue and gums. The microscopic lesions were characterized by hyperplasia of lymphoid cells at the haemopoietic centres in lymph glands and spleen followed by regression and degeneration of the germinal centres. Infiltration by lymphocytes and macrophages was observed in intermysial (heart) and periportal (liver) areas in interstitial spaces in kidneys. *T. annulata* parasitizes lymphoid cells. It provides stimulus for accelerated production of the cells which results in hyperplasia of the lymphoid tissue. Increased activity of the reticular tissue is a protective phenomenon in animals.

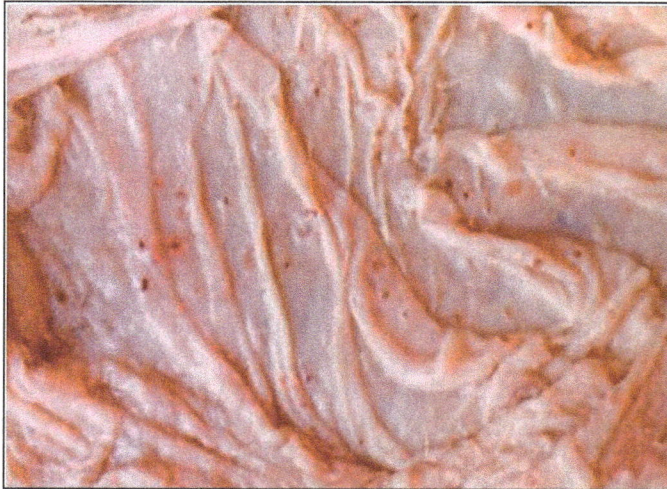

Figure 8: Theileriosis Infected Cattle Showing Ulcers in the Abomasum.

Babesiosis

Bovine babesiosis is also the most economically important disease because of direct loss on production.

Clinical Signs

Cattle with advanced babesiosis have a low exercise tolerance and sometimes collapse and die while being driven to a yard for treatment. Older animals are more acutely affected (clinical babesiosis is rare in cattle younger than six months). Abortions may occur when pregnant animals are severely affected. Similar clinical signs develop during infection with both organisms. However, the course of the disease differs markedly. Infections are characterised by:

1. Fever

2. Anorexia

3. Depression

4. Increased respiratory rate particularly following exertion

5. Muscle tremor

6. Reluctance to move

7. Haemoglobinuria

8. Occasionally signs of cerebral derangement such as circling, head pressing, mania and convulsions.

While these signs are seen very early in the course of *B. bovis* infections, they only develop in *B. bigemina* infections in the latter stages when parasitaemia is well advanced. Anaemia and jaundice develop steadily with *B. bovis*, but much more precipitously with *B. bigemina*. *B. bigemina* affected animals may exhibit irritability and aggression but not the central nervous system signs.

Clinical manifestations of disease associated with BB are typical of a haemolytic anaemia disease process but vary according to agent (*i.e.* species of parasite) and host factors (*i.e.* age, immune status). BB is predominantly observed in adult cattle with *B. bovis* generally being more pathogenic than *B. bigemina* or *B. divergens*. Infected animals develop a life-long immunity against re-infection with the same species and some cross-protection is evident in *B. bigemina*-immune animals against subsequent *B. bovis* infections.

Babesia bovis

1. High fever

2. Ataxia and incoordination

3. Anorexia

4. Production of dark red or brown-colored urine

5. Signs of general circulatory shock

6. Sometimes nervous signs associated with sequestration of infected erythrocytes in cerebral capillaries

7. In acute cases: maximum parasitaemia (percentage of infected erythrocytes) in circulating blood is often less than 1 per cent

Babesia bigemina

1. Fever

2. Haemoglobinuria and anaemia production of dark red or brown-colored urine

3. Nervous signs minimal or non-existent as intravascular sequestration of infected erythrocytes does not occur

4. Parasitaemia often exceeds 10 per cent and may be as high as 30 per cent

Babesia divergens

1. Parasitaemia and clinical appearance are similar to *B. bigemina* infections

Post-mortem Findings

Gross pathology seen in cases of babesiosis can be highly variable:

1. Varying degrees of congestion, pallor or jaundice
2. Blood is usually watery and urine is red
3. Sub-serosal haemorrhages are common, particularly on the heart and intestines
4. Spleen is enlarged with a soft red pulp
5. Liver is enlarged and brown or yellow, with the gall bladder filled with thick, granular bile

Lesions

1. Lesions observed are those most often associated with an intravascular haemolytic condition
2. Pale or icteric mucous membranes; blood may appear thin and watery
3. Subcutaneous tissues, abdominal fat and omentum may appear icteric
4. Swollen liver with an orange-brown or paler coloration; enlarged gall bladder containing thick, granular bile
5. Enlarged, dark, friable spleen
6. Kidneys appear darker than normal with possible petechial haemorrhages
7. Bladder may contain dark red or brown-colored urine
8. Possible oedema of lungs
9. Petechiae or ecchymoses on surface of heart and brain

Erhlichiosis and Anaplasmosis

Ruminants

Tick-borne fever occurs in domesticated ruminants, particularly sheep and cattle. It has also been documented in goats, deer and reindeer. In sheep, this disease is mainly seen in young lambs born in tick-infested areas, and in newly introduced older sheep. The primary syndrome is a sudden fever that lasts for 4 to 10 days. Other signs are generally mild and may include inappetance, weight loss or decreased weight gain, listlessness, coughing and increased respiratory and pulse rates. Abortions and stillbirths can occur in pregnant ewes introduced onto infected pastures during the last stages of gestation; abortions are usually seen 2 to 8 days after the onset of the fever. Semen quality can be significantly reduced in rams. In cattle, tick-borne fever usually occurs in dairy animals recently turned out to pasture. The clinical signs are variable in severity, but may include lethargy, marked anorexia, decreased milk production, coughing, respiratory distress, abortions, stillbirths and reduced semen quality. The two most prominent syndromes are abortions with a drop in milk yield and respiratory disease. In uncomplicated cases, animals usually recover within two weeks and deaths are uncommon except in aborting ewes. However, *A. phagocytophilum* increases the animal's susceptibility to other illnesses, which may be serious or fatal. Tick pyemia, caused by *Staphylococcus* spp., is the most frequent and severe complication in young lambs. This illness is characterized by severe lameness, debility and paralysis, and many lambs die. Pasteurellosis and septicemic listeriosis are also common complications.

Canine Ehrlichiosis and Anaplasmosis

The gross lesions are usually nonspecific in acute cases, but typically include enlargement of the spleen. Hemorrhagic lesions in severe canine ehrlichiosis can affect numerous organs including the gastrointestinal tract, heart, bladder, lungs, subcutaneous tissues and eyes. The lymph nodes, particularly the mesenteric nodes, may be enlarged, with red and brown discoloration on cut surface. There may be edema in the legs, as well as ascites and hydro pericardium. In chronic canine ehrlichiosis, splenomegaly and nonspecific lesions may be accompanied by widespread haemorrhages and microscopically by mononuclear cell infiltration into the perivascular area in multiple organs.

Equine Granulocytic Anaplasmosis

The characteristic lesions of equine granulocytic anaplasmosis are petechiae, ecchymoses and edema in the subcutaneous tissues and fascia, mainly in the legs. Interstitial pneumonitis has been reported in some animals.

Conclusions

It was concluded that body condition were very poor due to fever and anorexia that usually occur as a common clinical findings in cattle infected with theileriosis and babesiosis. However enlargement of lymph nodes and corneal opacity are associated clinical findings with theileriosis, while red brown to coffee urine and pale mucous membranes are associated clinical findings with babesiosis. Normocytic hypochromic anaemia is associated with theileriosis, while normocytic normochromic anaemia is associated with babesiosis. Phagocytic cells lymphocytes and monocytes are commonly increased in Theileria and Babesia infected cattle. Theileriosis and babesiosis have harmful effect on the liver function in cattle. Trypanosomiasis mostly occur in animals as carrier form and causes economic loss to the farmers.

Further Readings

1. Bal, M.S., Singla, L.D., Kumar, H, Vasudev, A., Gupta, K and Joyal, P.D. (2012). Pathological studies on experimental *Trypanosoma evansi* infection in Swiss albino mice. *J. Parasitic Diseases*, 36(2): 260-264.

2. Erhlichiosis and Anaplasomosis: zoonotic species, The Centre for food security and public health, Iowa State University, USA.

3. Sastry, G.A., 1983. *Veterinary Pathology*, CBS publishers and distributors, New Delhi, India. pp:685-692

Chapter 8

Enzyme-Linked Immunosorbent Assays in Disease Diagnosis

Rajeswari Shome

ICAR-National Institute of Veterinary Epidemiology and Disease Informatics (NIVEDI), Post Box No. 6450, Ramagondanahalli, Yelahanka, Bengaluru – 560 064, Karnataka

The Immuno enzymatic assay is the powerful laboratory technique for detection and measurement of variety of biological substance of clinical importance. This assay is a suitable alternative to the radioimmuno-assay due to its simplicity, requirement for relatively cheap and simple equipments, longer shelf life of its reagents and safety because of absence of radiation biohazards and disposable problems associated with radioactive waste. Enzyme-linked Immunosorbent Assays (ELISAs) is an immunoassay which combines the specificity of antibodies with the sensitivity of simple enzyme assays, by using antibodies or antigens coupled to an easily-assayed enzyme. The ELISA technique was conceptualized and developed by two Swedish scientists: Peter Perlmann (principal investigator) and Eva Engvall at Stockholm University in 1971.

ELISAs can provide a useful measurement of antigen or antibody concentration. There are two main variations on this method: The ELISA can be used to detect the presence of antigens that are recognized by an antibody or it can be used to test for antibodies that recognize an antigen. There are three necessary reagents: (a) antibody coupled to solid supports, "immunosorbent"; (b) antigen or antibody which is marked with enzyme and is called conjugate; (c) substrate.

According to the reagents, samples and the constitution of the detection, there are many different types of ELISAs, including the most common indirect ELISA, direct ELISA, sandwich ELISA, competitive ELISA, *etc.* According to different applications of ELISA, different types of ELISA can be chosen.

1. Direct ELISA

Direct ELISA, can be regarded as the simplest type of ELISA. In direct ELISA, an antigen is adsorbed to a plastic plate, then an excess of other protein (using bovine serum albumin) is added to block all the other binding sites. Then an enzyme is linked to an antibody in a separate reaction. The enzyme-antibody conjugate is allowed to adsorb to the antigen, then excess enzyme-antibody conjugate is washed off, leaving enzyme-antibody bound to antigen. By adding the enzyme's substrate, the enzyme is detected and thus the antigen.

2. Indirect ELISA

Indirect ELISA, the steps are similar, but with important differences and an additional step. After the antigen is adsorbed to the plate, the next antibody to be added is the antibody that recognizes the antigen (this antibody does not have the enzyme attached to it). Then, an enzyme-antibody conjugate is prepared, which is added to the plate and detects the antibody that is adsorbed to the antigen, then the substrate is added which detects the presence of the enzyme and thus the antigen.

e.g.: Detection of antibodies against *Besnoitia besnoiti* in cattle serum or plasma.

3. Competitive ELISA

This is another variation for measurement of antigen. After addition of the primary antibody unlabelled sample containing antigen is added.Upon addition of conjugated antigen followed by substrate colour change is observed if the conjugated Ag bind to the sites of the primary antibody which are not occupied by unlabelled antigen. The concentration of antigen is inversely proportional to the colour produced so more the unlabelled antigen in the sample lesser the amount of conjugated antigen bound.

e.g.: Antibody detection of various parasitic diseases.

4. Sandwich ELISA

The plate is coated with a capture antibody followed by the addition of sample. The antigen present will bind to capture antibody. Then the detecting antibody is added, which binds to the antigen. This is followed by the addition of enzyme-linked secondary antibody which will bind to detecting antibody, and then the substrate is added, and is converted by enzyme to detectable form.

e.g.: Detection of Antibodies to Porcine Circovirus 2, detection of antigen of foot-and-mouth disease virus (FMDV), Equine encephalosis virus, Newcastle Disease Virus, Peste des petits ruminant in sheep and goats.

Use of monoclonal antibodies in Competitive and Sandwich ELISA systems

☆ **Higher sensitivity** : either by selection of antibodies with a extremely high affinity, or by reduction of the height and variability of the background reaction, which makes very low concentrations of analyte more readily detectable.

☆ **Higher specificity** : by avoiding the presence of any antibody in the assay system with specific reactivity against non-analyte epitopes, and by selecting combinations of monoclonal antibodies which may further increase specificity.

☆ **Higher practicality** : *e.g.* by introducing simultaneous incubation of label, solid phase and sample without risk of "prozone effect".

5. Avidin-Biotin Complex (ABC) ELISA Method

This test includes a secondary antibody coupled to biotin molecule following which the Avidin Biotin peroxidase complex added. The substrate on being reacted by the enzyme produces the color. In the test the Avidin molecules serves as a bridge between the biotin molecules and since the Avidin has four biotin binding sites the signal observed by the technique is approximately four times that of normal ELISA. It can detect very low level of antibodies in serum.

e.g.: detection of parasitic disease antigen.

Enzymes and Substrates Used in ELISA

Most of the assays employ horse-radish peroxidase, alkaline phosphatase, or B-D-galactosidase. The most interesting recent developments have been in new methods to detect these enzymes rather than the use of new enzymes. Fluorimeters were introduced in 1984 for the detection of alkaline phosphatase and B-D-galactosidase. Methods are available to detect horse radish peroxidase by means of chemilumininescence. Fluorimetric and luminometric methods offer higher sensitivity and a wider measuring range than conventional spectrometry. TMB is gradually replacing mutagenic substrates such as OPD, leading to increased sensitivity and safety.

Enzyme	*Substrate*	*Colour*
Horseradish Peroxidase (HRP)	(TMB)	Blue (652nm)
	(OPD)	Yellow (492nm)
	(ABTS)	Green (410nm)
β-Galactosidase	o-Nitrophenyle-β-D-galactopyranosite (ONPG)	Yellow (405nm)
Alkaline Phosphatase	P-nitro phenyl phosphate (PNPP)	Yellow (405nm)

Advantages of ELISA

☆ Fast- 90 samples tested in 2-3 hr

☆ High Sensitivity (up to 10 pg/mL)

☆ Strong Specificity

☆ Many samples can be processed at once

☆ Small sample size required (10 µL~ 100µL)

✰ Colorimetric results –easily observed and measured(spectrophotometer)

✰ Test for presence of Ag or Ab

✰ Flexible usage for research design

✰ Easy to learn, simple procedure

Disadvantages of ELISA

✰ Negative controls may indicate positive results if blocking solution is ineffective [secondary antibody or antigen (unknown sample) can bind to open sites in well]

✰ Enzyme/substrate reaction is short term so microwells must be read as soon as possible

✰ Monoclonal antibodies can cost more than polyclonal antibodies

✰ Test requires sophisticated instruments like ELISA reader to read the results

✰ Cannot be used under field condition

Application of ELISA

✰ ELISA is used as an alternative tool for epidemiological surveillance.

✰ Disease outbreaks- tracking the spread of disease.

✰ Serum Antibody Concentrations.

✰ Detections of antigens.

✰ Detection of antibodies in blood sample for past exposure to disease.

Trouble Shooting Tips in ELISA

Background Color

Background color in the plate can be minimized by proper washing or by using higher dilution of conjugate and also by reducing the incubation temperature of the conjugate. Substrate incubation carried out in light and also plate left too long before reading on incubation time on the plate reader also leads to background color.

Positive Results in Negative Control

May be contamination of reagents or samples, Insufficient washing of plates, too much antibody used leading to non-specific binding and also contaminants from laboratory glassware like antibodies, peroxides can also gives the false positive results.

Low Absorbance Values

Insufficient antibody, substrate solutions not fresh or combined incorrectly, Reagents not fresh or not at the correct pH, Incubation time not long enough, Incubation temperature too low, stop solution not added all these conditions will lead to low absorbance values.

High Absorbance Values for Samples and/or Positive Control

Reduce the concentration of samples and control by dilution before adding to the plate. Take the dilution into account when calculating the resulting concentrations.

Color Developing Slowly

Plates are not at the correct temperature or maybe because of too weak conjugate. Presence of contaminants, such as sodium azide and peroxidise can affect the substrate reaction.

Improper Antigen Binding

Prefer polysorp plates if the antigen nature is hydrophobic and Maxisorb/High binding p plates if the protein nature is unknown.

Further Reading

1. Jacobson, R.H. (1998). Validation of serological assays for diagnosis of infectious diseases. *Rev. Sci. Tech.* 17, 469–486.

Chapter 9

Polymerase Chain Reaction (PCR): Principle and its Application in Disease Diagnosis

V. Balamurugan, M. Nagalingam and D.S.N. Raju

*ICAR-National Institute of Veterinary Epidemiology and
Disease Informatics (NIVEDI), Post Box No. 6450,
Ramagondanahalli, Yelahanka, Bengaluru – 560 064, Karnataka*

Polymerase chain reaction (PCR) is a molecular technique to amplify a single or a few copies of a piece of DNA across several orders of magnitude, generating thousands to millions of copies of a particular DNA sequence. The method relies on thermal cycling, consisting of cycles of repeated heating and cooling of the reaction for DNA melting and enzymatic replication of the DNA. Primers (short DNA fragments) containing sequences complementary to the target region along with a DNA polymerase are key components to enable selective and repeated amplification. As PCR progresses, the DNA generated is itself used as a template for replication, setting in motion a chain reaction in which the DNA template is exponentially amplified. The steps involved are denaturation, annealing and extension followed by final extension to complete the products length.PCR was invented in 1984 by Dr. Kary Banks Mullis and he received the Nobel Prize in chemistry in 1993, for his invention.

The following are the different phases in PCR assay. *Exponential phase:* If 100 per cent efficiency–exact doubling of products have been taken place that is very specific and recise. *Linear Phase*: High variability. Reaction components are being consumed and PCR products are starting to degrade. *Plateau phase:* End-point analysis. The reaction has stopped and if left for long, degradation of PCR products will begin.

Primers

Each primer should be 20-30 nucleotides in length and contain approximately equal number of four bases (A, T, G and C) with a balanced distribution of G and C residues and a low propensity to form stable secondary structures. Primers can be designed manually or using softwares (Eg DNASTAR, Primer3 *etc.*,). Standard reactions contain non limiting amount of primers, typically 0.1-0.5 µM of each primer.

Template DNA

DNA can be extracted from Whole blood of livestock using conventional method or Blood genomic extraction kit. The blood is collected using EDTA vacutainers.

Deoxynucleoside Triphosphates (dNTPs)

Standard PCRs contain equimolar amounts of dATP, dTTP, dCTP and dGTP. Concentrations of 200-250 µM of each dNTP are recommended for reaction containing 1.5mM $MgCl_2$.

DNA Polymerase

A thermostable DNA polymerase, routinely *Taq* polymerase is used to catalyse template-dependent synthesis of DNA. Usually 0.5 to 2.5 units per standard 25-50 µl reaction is used.

Real-time PCR Assay

The most powerful tool for quantitative nucleic acid analysis is the real-time PCR, which is a refinement of the original PCR developed in the mid-1980 and found useful for medical and scientific arena in diagnostic applications (Kubista *et al.*, 2006). In real-time PCR, the amount of product formed is monitored during the course of the reaction by monitoring the fluorescence of dyes or probes incorporated into the reaction that is proportional to the amount of product formed, and the number of amplification cycles required to obtain a particular amount of DNA molecules is registered. In conventional PCR, the amplified product, or amplicon, is detected by an end-point analysis, by running DNA on an agarose gel after the reaction has finished. In contrast, real-time PCR allows the accumulation of amplified product to be detected and measured as the reaction progresses, that is, in "real-time". Real-time detection of PCR products is made possible by including in the reaction a fluorescent molecule that reports an increase in the amount of DNA with a proportional increase in fluorescent signal. The fluorescent chemistries employed for this purpose include DNA-binding dyes and fluorescently labeled sequence-specific primers or probes. Specialized thermal cyclers equipped with fluorescence detection modules are used to monitor the fluorescence as amplification occurs. The measured fluorescence reflects the amount of amplified product in each cycle. Real-time PCR has the ability to directly measure the PCR reaction as amplification is taking place with the use of fluorescent molecules.

Principle of real-time is based on the detection and quantitation of a fluorescent reporter. Three general methods for the quantitative detection by using 1. DNA-binding dyes/agents (SYBR Green), 2. Hydrolysis probes (TaqMan, Beacons, Scorpions), 3. Hybridisation probes (Light Cycler). Others Includes, Dye-labeled, sequence-specific oligonucleotide primers or probes (molecular beacons and TaqMan, hybridization, and Eclipse probes, and Amplifluor, Scorpions, LUX, and BD QZyme primers, *etc.*).

RT_PCR Chemistry

The most commonly used chemistries for real-time PCR are the DNA-binding dye SYBR Green I and TaqMan hydrolysis probes. In real-time PCR, DNA binding dyes are used as fluorescent reporters to monitor the real-time PCR reaction. If a graph is drawn between the log of the starting amount of template and the corresponding increase the fluorescence of the reporter dye fluorescence during real-time PCR, a linear relationship is observed. Based on the molecule used for the detection, the real-time PCR techniques can be categorically placed under two heads namely non-specific detection using DNA binding dyes and specific detection target specific probes.

Advantages of Real-Time PCR

☆ Not influenced by non-specific amplification

☆ Amplification can be monitored real-time

☆ No post-PCR processing of products (high throughput, low contamination risk)

☆ Ultra-rapid cycling (30 minutes to 2 hours)

☆ Wider dynamic range of up to 1010 fold

☆ Detection is capable down to a 2-fold change

☆ Confirmation of specific amplification by melting point analysis

☆ Not much more expensive than conventional PCR

Disadvantages of Real-Time PCR

☆ Not ideal for multiplexing in general

☆ Setting up requires high technical skill and support

☆ High equipment cost

☆ Intra- and inter-assay variation

☆ RNA lability

☆ DNA contamination (in mRNA analysis)

Application of Real-Time PCR

Typical uses of real-time PCR include pathogen detection, gene expression analysis, single nucleotide polymorphism (SNP) analysis, analysis of chromosome aberrations, and most recently protein detection by real-time immuno-PCR has also been reported (Kubista *et al.*, 2006). Real-time PCR is used to quantitate DNA or RNA samples. Real-time PCR is the most accurate method to detect copy number of each gene, amount of gene expression, efficiency of drugs, Bacterial/Virus infection, different type of pathogens, methylation of DNA, different type of mutations, adverse effect of organ transplantation *etc.,*

Further Readings

1. Kubista M, Andrade J M, Bengtsson M., *et al.* (2006).The real-time polymerase chain reaction. *Mol. Aspects. Med.* **2-3**:95-125.

2. Molecular Cloning: A Laboratory Manual (Third Edition) by Joseph Sambrook, Peter MacCallum Cancer Institute, Melbourne, Australia; David Russell, University of Texas Southwestern Medical Center, Dallas.

Chapter 10

Real-time PCR in Animal Disease Diagnosis

B.R. Shome and Susweta Das Mitra

ICAR-National Institute of Veterinary Epidemiology and
Disease Informatics (NIVEDI), Post Box No. 6450,
Ramagondanahalli, Yelahanka, Bengaluru – 560 064, Karnataka

Making an accurate diagnosis of disease contributes to both the characterization of disease epidemiology and to individual animal care (Thaipadunpanit *et al.*, 2011). In recent years, quantitative real-time PCR tests have been extensively developed in clinical microbiology laboratories for routine diagnosis of infectious diseases (Max Maurin 2012)

Real-time PCR is a laboratory technique of molecular biology based on the polymerase chain reaction (PCR), which is used to amplify and simultaneously quantify a targeted DNA molecule. The quantity can be either an absolute number of copies or a relative amount when normalized to DNA input or additional normalizing genes.

General Principle

The procedure follows the general principle of polymerase chain reaction; its key feature is that the amplified DNA is detected as the reaction progresses in "real-time". This is a new approach compared to standard PCR, where the product of the reaction is detected at its end. Two common methods for the detection of products in quantitative PCR (Max Maurin 2012) are:

Chemistry used-Real-time PCR Technology

1. SYBR® Green assay: The first using a fluorescent dye, such as SYBR® Green, which binds nonspecifically to double stranded DNA, where the

resulting DNA–dye complex absorbs blue light (l_{max} = 497 nm) and emits green light (l_{max} = 520 nm) detected by the qPCR instrument. SYBR Green and dual-hybridization probes are often used for melting point analysis at the end of the amplification.

(ii) PROBE assay: The second using fluorescent resonance energy transfer (FRET) probes, which bind specifically to the amplified DNA. The sequence-specific DNA probes consisting of oligonucleotides that are labelled with a fluorescent reporter permits detection only after hybridization of the probe with its complementary sequence to quantify messenger RNA (mRNA) and non-coding RNA in cells or tissues.

The term FRET probe refers to a generic mechanism in which emission/ quenching relies on the interaction between the electron-excitation states of two fluorescent dye molecules. Different FRET probes exist, including 52-nuclease probes (also named hydrolysis or TaqMan® probes), dual-hybridization probes (also named LightCycler® probes), molecular beacons and scorpion probes.

Diagnostic Uses

There are numerous applications for quantitative polymerase chain reaction in the laboratory. It is commonly used for both diagnostic and basic research. Diagnostic quantitative PCR is applied to rapidly detect nucleic acids that are diagnostic of, for example, infectious diseases, cancer and genetic abnormalities. The introduction of quantitative PCR assays to the clinical microbiology laboratory has significantly improved the diagnosis of infectious diseases,[29] and is deployed as a tool to detect newly emerging diseases.

Quantification Strategies

The quantification strategy is the principal marker in gene quantification. Generally two strategies can be performed in real-time RT-PCR. The levels of expressed genes may be measured by absolute or relative quantitative real-time RT-PCR (Figure 9, Table 1).

(i) Absolute Quantification

Absolute quantification relates the PCR signal to input copy number using a calibration curve, while relative quantification measures the relative change in mRNA expression levels. The reliability of an absolute real-time RT-PCR assay depends on the condition of 'identical' amplification efficiencies for both the native target and the calibration curve in RT reaction and in following kinetic PCR.

(ii) Relative Quantification

Relative quantification is easier to perform than absolute quantification because a calibration curve is not necessary. It is based on the expression levels of a target gene versus a housekeeping gene (reference or control gene) and in theory is adequate for most purposes to investigate physiological changes in gene expression levels. The units used to express relative quantities are irrelevant, and the relative quantities can be compared across multiple real-time RT-PCR experiments.

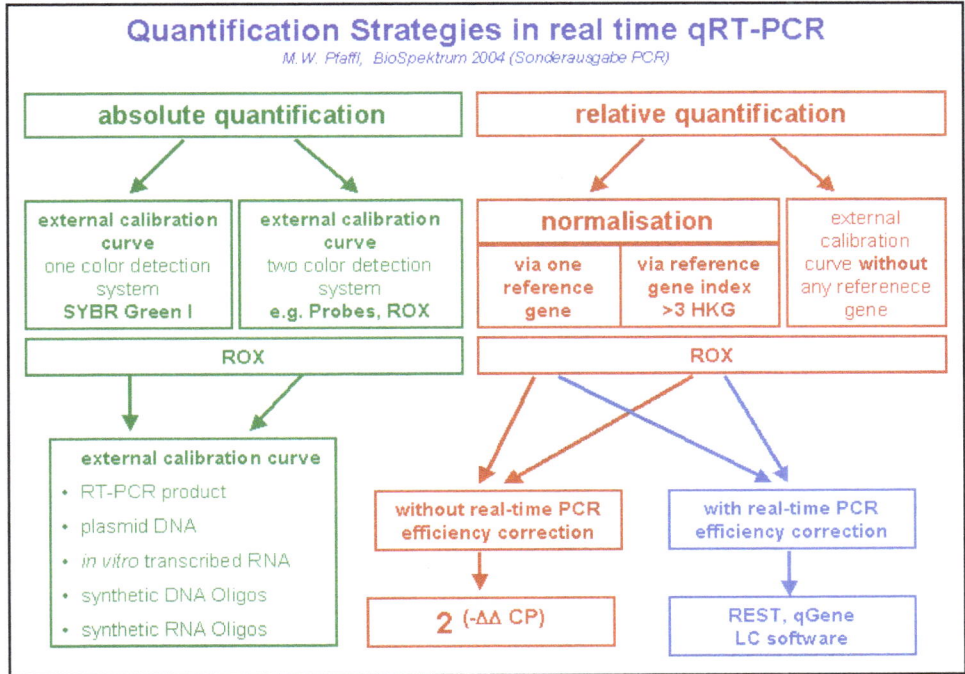

Figure 9: Quantification Strategies in Real-Time qRT PCR.

Table 1: Absolute vs Relative Quantification at a Glance

	Absolute Quantification (Digital PCR Method)	Absolute Quantification (Standard Curve Method)	Relative Quantification
Overview	In absolute quantification using Digital PCR, no known standards are needed. The target of interest can be directly quantified with precision determined by number of digital PCR replicates.	In absolute quantification using the Standard Curve Method, you quantitate unknowns based on a known quantity. First you create a standard curve; then you compare unknowns to the standard curve and extrapolate a value.	In relative quantification, you analyze changes in gene expression in a given sample relative to another reference sample (such as an untreated control sample).
Example	Quantify copies of rare allele present in heterogenous mixtures. Count the number of cell equivalents in sample by targeting genomic DNA. Determine absolute number of viral copies present in a given sample without reference to a standard.	Correlating viral copy number with a disease state.	Measuring gene expression in response to a drug. In this example, you would compare the level of gene expression of a particular gene of interest in a chemically treated sample relative to the level of gene expression in an untreated sample.

Laboratory Protocol

(i) SYBR Green Assay

Generation of PCR products can be detected by measurement of the SYBR Green I Fluorescence signal. SYBR Green I intercalates into the DNA helix. In solution the unbound dye exhibits very little fluorescence, however fluorescence (Wavelength 530 nm) is greatly enhanced upon DNA binding. Therefore during PCR, the increase in SYBR Green I fluorescence is directly proportional to the amount of double stranded DNA generated.

The following protocol is for Light Cycler480 real-time system:

Sample Material

Template DNA (*e.g.* Genomic or Plasmid DNA, cDNA) suitable for PCR in terms of purity, concentration, and absence of inhibitors). Use upto 50-100ng complex genomic DNA or up to 10^8 copies plasmid DNA for reaction volume of 20 µl.

Materials and Equipments

- ☆ Real-time PCR analysis system
- ☆ Multi well Plate 96
- ☆ Swing bucket centrifuge containing a rotor for multiwall plates with suitable adapters
- ☆ Bench top centrifuge for 1.5mL Eppendorf tubes
- ☆ Nuclease free, aerosol-resistant pipette tips and
- ☆ Pipettes (range 10, 200, 1000µL) with disposable, positive displacement tips
- ☆ Sterile reaction (Eppendorf) tubes for preparing master mixes and dilutions
- ☆ Light Cycler 480 SYBR Green I Master kit
- ☆ The specific primers and probes for the target genes

Preparation of PCR Master Mix (LC480 SYBR Green I master KIT)

Procedure to Prepare one 20µl Standard Reaction

- ☆ Do not touch the surface of the Light Cycler 480 Multiwell Plate and Multiwell Sealing Foil when handling them. Always wear gloves during handling.
- ☆ Thaw one vial of Light Cycler 480 SYBR Green I Master (vial 1, green cap) and Water, PCR Grade. (Keep the Master Mix away from light).
- ☆ Prepare a 10X conc. Solution of the PCR primers
- ☆ In a 1.5 ml reaction tube on ice, prepare the PCR Mix for one 20 µl reaction by adding the following components in the order mentioned below:

Component	Volume
Water, PCR-grade (vial 2, colorless cap)	4 µl
Forward Primer (5picomole/µl)	2 µl
Reverse Primer, (5picomole/µl)	2 µl
Master Mix 2x conc. (vial 1, Green cap)	10 µl
Total volume	18
To prepare the PCR mix for more than one reaction, multiply the amount in the "Volume" column above by Y, where Y= the number of reactions to be run)	

☆ Mix carefully by pipe ting up and down. Do not vortex.

☆ Pipette 18 µl PCR mix into each well of the Multiwell Plate

☆ Add 2 µl of the DNA template

☆ Seal the multiwall plate with Multiwell Sealing foil

☆ Place the Multiwell Plate in the centrifuge and balance it with a suitable counterweight (*e.g.* Another Multiwell Plate) Centrifuge at 1500x g for 2 mins.

☆ Load the Multiwell Plate into the Real-time (Light Cycler) Instrument

☆ Start the PCR program as described below

Instrument Protocol

Table shows the PCR parameters that must be programmed into the Real-time Instrument

Detection Format	Block type	Reaction Volume
SYBR Green	96	10-100µl
PROGRAMS		
Program name	Cycles	Analysis Mode
(i) Pre-incubation	1	None
(ii) Amplification	40	Quantification
(iii) Cooling	1	None
TEMPERATURE TARGETS		
Pre-incubation		
95ºC	00:05:00	
Amplification		
95ºC	00:00:10	
60ºC (primer dependent)	00:00:10	
72ºC	00:00:30	
Melting Curve		
95ºC	00:00:05	
60ºC	00:01:00	
95ºC	Continuous	
Cooling		
40ºC	00:00:10	

(ii) PROBE Assay

LightCycler® 480 Probes Master is designed for real-time PCR using the LightCycler® 480 Instrument in combination with suitable probes (*e.g.*, hydrolysis probes, Universal ProbeLibrary probes, and others) and gene-specific primers. The kit is ideally suited for hot-start PCR assays for gene quantification and Endpoint Genotyping assays.

Preparation of the PCR mix (Light Cycler 480 Probes Master kit)

Do not touch the surface of the Light Cycler 480 Multiwell Plate and Multiwell Sealing Foil when handling them. Always wear gloves during handling.

1. Thaw the solutions and to ensure recovery of all contents, briefly spin vials in a micro centrifuge before opening
2. Mix carefully by pipetting up and down and store in ice.
3. Prepare a 5 pico moles/µl solution of the PCR primers
4. In a 1.5 ml reaction tube on ice, prepare the PCR Mix for one 20 µl reaction by adding the following components in the order mentioned below:

Component	Volume
Water, PCR-grade (vial 2, colorless cap)	3.8 µl
Gene specific	2 µl
Forward Primer (5picomole/µl)	
Reverse Primer (5picomole/µl)	2 µl
Probe 0.2 µM	0.2 µl
Master Mix 2x conc. (vial 1, Green cap)	10 µl
Total volume	18
To prepare the PCR mix for more than one reaction, multiply the amount in the "Volume" column above by Y, where Y= the number of reactions to be run)	

5. Mix carefully by pipetting up and down. Do not vortex.
6. Pipette 18 µl PCR mix into each well of the Multiwell Plate
7. Add 2 µl of the DNA template
8. Seal the multiwall plate with Multiwell Sealing foil
9. Place the Multiwell Plate in the centrifuge and balance it with a suitable counterweight (*e.g.* Another Multiwell Plate) Centrifuge at 1500x g for 2 mins.
10. Load the Multiwell Plate into the Real-time (Light Cycler) Instrument
11. Start the PCR program as described below

Instrument Protocol

The Table shows the PCR parameters that must be programmed into the Light Cycler 480 Real-time Instrument with the Light Cycler 480 Probes Master (kit) using LC 480 Multiwell Plate 96.

PCR Parameters

Detection Format	Block type	Reaction Volume
Mono Color Hydrolysis Probes	96	10-100µl
PROGRAMS		
Program name	Cycles	Analysis Mode
(i) Pre-incubation	1	None
(ii) Amplification	40	Quantification
(iii) Cooling	1	None
TEMPERATURE TARGETS		
Pre-incubation		
95ºC	00:05:00	
Amplification		
95ºC	00:00:10	
60ºC (primer dependent)	00:00:10	
72ºC	00:00:30	
Cooling		
40ºC	00:00:10	

Data analysis

The data obtained from real-time RT-PCR analysis are Cycle Threshold (CT) values that are a measure of the amount of starting target material (Fig 2). The CT values need to be converted using different procedures to make valid comparisons. When conducting a real-time PCR experiment that uses an absolute quantification procedure, it is necessary to compare the CT value for each sample with the standard curve. After locating the CT value on the standard curve, one will have a measurement that corresponds to the copy number (or amount) of the target sequence in the starting template sample.

Absolute quantification: For Absolute Quantification analyses, serial dilutions of an external standard with predefined known concentration are used to create a standard curve. The standard dilutions are amplified in separate wells but within the same Light Cycler® 480 Instrument run. The crossing points of standards and unknown samples are then used to determine the concentration of target DNA.

LC480 provides two methods for performing Absolute Quantification analysis

☆ Second Derivative Maximum method

☆ Fit Points method.

Both methods use standard curves to calculate unknown sample concentrations, but each method determines a sample's crossing point in a different way (LightCycler® 480 Instrument Operator's Manual Software Version 1.5).

Relative quantification: On the other hand relative quantification compares the levels of two different target sequences in a single sample (*e.g.*, target gene of

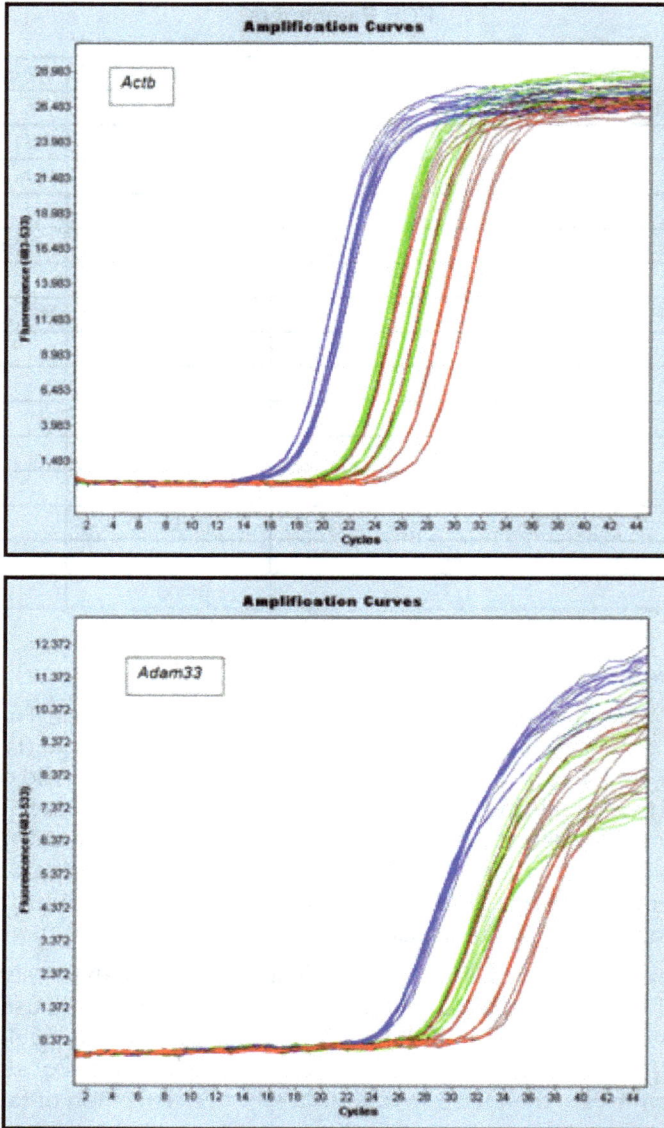

Figure 10: Amplification Curves for Genes. Y-axis is the change in fluorescence and x-axis is the PCR cycle number (Cp value).

interest (GOI) and another gene) and expresses the final result as a ratio of these targets. For comparison purposes the second gene is a reference gene that is found in constant copy numbers under all test conditions. This reference gene, which is also known as endogenous control, provides a basis for normalizing sample-to sample differences. The versatile Light Cycler® 480 Relative Quantification Software provides different relative quantification methods (*e.g.,* basic CT-Method, advanced E-Method with standard-curve derived efficiencies) for gene expression studies.

Further Readings

1. Sails AD (2009)."Applications in Clinical Microbiology". Real-Time PCR: Current Technology and Applications. Caister Academic Press. ISBN 978-1-904455-39-4.

2. Thaipadunpanit J, Chierakul W, Wuthiekanun V, Limmathurotsakul D, Amornchai P, *et al.* (2011). Diagnostic Accuracy of Real-Time PCR Assays Targeting 16S rRNA and lipl32 Genes for Human Leptospirosis in Thailand: A Case-Control Study. *PLoS ONE* 6(1): e16236. doi:10.1371/journal.pone.0016236.

3. Max Maurin (2012). Real-time PCR as a Diagnostic Tool for Bacterial Diseases. *Expert Rev Mol Diagn*. 12: 731-754.

4. Fouchier, R. M., Bestebroer, T. M., Herfst S., Vanderkemp L., *et al.* (2000). Detection of Inuenza A Viruses from Different Species by PCR. *Journal of Clini Microbiol.*, 38: 4096-4101

5. LightCycler® 480 Instrument Operator's Manual Software Version 1.5 http:// icob.sinica.edu.tw/pubweb/Core per cent 20Facilities/Data/R401-core/ LightCycler480 per cent 20II_Manual_V1.5.pdf.

Chapter 11

Novel Biotechnological Tools for Diagnosis and Control of Blood Protozoal Diseases in Animals

M. Nagalingam, V. Balamurugan and R. Shome

ICAR-National Institute of Veterinary Epidemiology and
Disease Informatics (NIVEDI), Post Box No. 6450,
Ramagondanahalli, Yelahanka, Bengaluru – 560 064, Karnataka

Parasites play a major role in causing diseases of man and livestock. They attribute to the major economic loss in the animal husbandry sector. A possible solution to these problems lies in the development of new technologies to suit expanding livestock sector. One of the ways in which livestock production can be increased is by reduction of losses due to disease. Few reports estimate that only a 6 per cent reduction in disease could provide food for an additional 250 million people. The value of biotechnology-based products for use in animal health was US$ 2.8 billion in 2007 (OIE, 2007) and the veterinary vaccines contribution to this global market was approximately 23 per cent. In the last thirty years there has been a shift of focus in dealing with clinical diseases from treatment aspect to prophylactic disease prevention. In the future, diagnostics and vaccines are expected to bring in more impact and income compared to pharmaceuticals in the livestock sector.

Novel Biotechnological Tools in Diagnosis

Identification of the organism is the most assured way to diagnose a parasitic infection. Laboratory diagnosis plays vital role in the evaluation of the disease process, either confirming a presumptive diagnosis or giving evidence of disease. However, possibility of infection is not excluded whenever there is failure to demonstrate or recover a parasite. By microscopic examination, many of the parasites, mainly the protozoa, can be identified. Other methods relied on detecting antibodies by agar gel immunodiffusion (AGID), complement xation (CFT) and enzyme-linked immunosorbent assay (ELISA). In the past thirty years, molecular techniques such as PCR and its variants, western blot, recombinant proteins, monoclonal antibodies and synthetic peptides have been incorporated in the diagnostics. Although conventional diagnostic assays are still widely used, new biotechnological techniques have improved the scope in veterinary diagnostics and provide robust new tools that enable the sensitive and specic diagnosis of animal diseases.

Advances in Immunoassays

Immunoassays are based on the principle of the affinity binding between antibodies and the respective antigen resulting in detection of either antigen or antibody in blood, serum, milk, CSF and other biological fluids. Radio labeled immunoassays (RIA) were developed initially which used radioisotopes to detect free and bound antigen. Although RIAs are good at sensitivity, the biohazard nature of radioisotopes made them to get replaced by many other assays or approaches.

1. **Fluorescence**: Fluorescent label is tagged to antibodies, so that they can be applied directly to tissue sections which can be observed under microscope for detection of antigens *e.g.*immuno histo chemistry. The limitation may include photo bleaching.

2. **Enzyme**: Enzyme conjugate is linked to an antibody so that it produces coloured reaction when added with substrate and the absorbance (optical density) is measured using spectrophotometry. This technique called ELISA is being used in many of the diagnostic tests aimed to detect antibodies. However they are used for detecting antigens also. Many of the variants include Direct, Indirect, Competitive, Sandwich ELISA *etc.*, Dip stick assays are also based on similar approach.

3. **Chemiluminescence**: Measures emission of light as a result of chemical reaction (antigen-antibody aggregation).

4. **Light scattering**: Measures the light scattering produced by aggregates of antigen and antibody.

5. **Electrochemical tags**: Measures the redox potential by measuring current.

Advanced molecular tools such as recombinant DNA technology, peptide synthesis, antibody engineering have made possible the synthesis of specific protein which can act as an epitope or antigen or antibody to be used in diagnostic assays. Synthetic peptides can be used as positive control which avoids the handling of pathogenic organisms. In cases where particular pathogen is eliminated using control programs, it becomes difficult to handle the organism to extract antigen to be used in the diagnostics and synthetic peptides or recombinant antigens provide an alternative solution. Since animal origin materials such as eggs or fetal bovine serum may contain unexpected or cross reacting antigens which may affect the downstream processing, transgenic plants expressing veterinary pathogen proteins offer an excellent and effective method of making large amounts of recombinant proteins.

Generally diagnostic assays are performed in laboratories where infra structure and relevant equipments are available. Often pen side or field side diagnostics can offer timely and low cost solution for effective and efficient intervention. The assays can be aimed at detecting antigen or antibody. One such assay is lateral flow assay where in serum or milk to be added with diluent and put at one end. The membrane allows the migration of the sample based on capillary action and the principle is more or less similar to ELISA. As the sample migrates each step of ELISA occurs sequentially and finally if the analyte is present it develops a coloured line. These assays usually provide a qualitative result. These assay formats in addition to their simplicity, they don't require electricity, skilled technicians, sophisticated equipments *etc.*, Recent advances leading to palm held Fluorescent Polarization Assay (FPA) instruments, portable PCR machines and ELISA readers are bringing lab to the pen side.

Biosensors

Biosensor is a compact analytical device based upon a transducer with a bio recognition element able to transform a biochemical event on the transducer into a measurable signal. Biosensors are directed towards detection of either antigen or antibody. The earliest biosensors were catalytic systems followed by affinity biosensors. The transducers used are electrochemical, thermometric, optical, magnetic and piezoelectric. Nucleic acid-based biosensors in which oligonucleotide either integrated within or intimately linked with a signal transducer, can be used to detect DNA/RNA fragments. Use of antibodies in multi-analyte detection method could face some limitations, aptamers which are single-stranded DNA or RNA against amino acids, proteins, drugs, and other molecules are being used in biosensors. Biosensors are mostly linked with sophisticated instrumentation to produce highly-specic analytical results. Due to the high cost, most of them are limited only to research. It also requires highly skilled technicians. Immuno sensors have been used for the diagnosis of anaplasmosis.

Detection of Nucleic Acids

In veterinary medicine, the use of nucleic acid-based diagnostics has increased exponentially in recent years. These techniques have redefined the level of information available for animal disease control programmes. The techniques include

1. *Nucleic acid extraction:* A basic and important step in the molecular diagnostic procedure is extraction of 'pure' nucleic acid mixtures to act as a template for further reactions.

2. *Polymerase chain reaction (PCR) and real-time PCR:* The molecular technique with the greatest variety and use in veterinary diagnostics is PCR. There are many variations of PCR such as Hot-start PCR, RT-PCR, Inverse PCR, Multiplex PCR, AFLP PCR, Nested PCR, Asymmetric PCR, Competitive PCR, Ligation-mediated PCR, Assembly PCR, and also the real-time PCR.

Techniques have been developed for fast diagnosis of bovine theileriosis by whole blood PCR followed by microchip electrophoresis.

3. *Isothermal amplification:* These technologies are advantageous which enable DNA amplification at constant temperature by omitting thermo cycling.

   i. Loop-mediated isothermal amplification (LAMP)-It is practiced widely which employs two sets of specially designed primers forming a stem-loop DNA by self-primed DNA synthesis and a DNA polymerase (*Bst* polymerase) having strand displacement activity. The amplification process produces loops at the ends of the complementary strands, which are extended continually. The amplification is confirmed by either the appearance of turbidity (pyrophosphate byproducts form a white precipitate that increases the turbidity) or using fluorescent dyes resulting in generation of fluorescent signal. The detection of amplification products can be by various other methods including electrophoretic, electrochemical and turbidimetric

   ii. Isothermal multiple displacement amplification (IMDA) - This reaction utilizes random hexamers with Phi 29 DNA polymerase.

   iii. Ligase chain reaction (LCR)-It amplifies nucleic acid as the probe. DNA polymerase and DNA ligase were used in this reaction.

   iv. Transcription-mediated amplification (TMA) – RNA polymerase and reverse transcriptase are used to amplify target RNA or DNA.

   v. Signal-mediated amplification of RNA technology (SMART)- It produces target-dependent multiple copies of an RNA signal, and measured by an enzyme-linked oligosorbent assay.

   vi. Nucleic acid sequence-based amplification (NASBA)-Amplification of RNA sequences using reverse transcriptase, RNase H and RNA polymerase. NASBA based diagnostic has been developed for the diagnosis of *Trypanosoma brucei*.

   vii. Strand displacement amplification (SDA) - Use of HincII and exonuclease deficient klenow for nucleic acid amplification.

   viii. Self-sustained sequence replication (3SR)- Amplification using reverse transcriptase, RNase H and RNA polymerase and can be coupled directly to in vitro translation systems

   ix. Helicase-dependent amplification (HDA) - DNA helicase separates double stranded DNA and single stranded DNA (ssDNA)-binding proteins help them to remain separated so that two sequence specific primers hybridise to each and DNA polymerase produce a double stranded DNA.

   x. Strand invasion-based amplification (SIBA) - Insertion of an invasion oligo into the double stranded nucleic acid and polymerase will extend the primers.

   xi. recombinase polymerase amplification (RPA) - It employs recombinase, SSB protein and strand-displacing polymerase for the amplification.

xii. Ramification amplification method (RAM)- uses circular probe (C-probe) in which the 3' and 5' ends are brought together by hybridization to a target and polymerase amplifies in rolling circle model.

4. *Nucleic acid detection without amplification-* Surface-enhanced Raman scattering (SERS) has led to a new approach for detection of target DNA. The method is based on capturing a thiol-conjugated probe and a reporter probe labeled with methylene blue, which are linked to the target complementary DNA. A Raman label places the methylene blue on a gold or silver nano particle, to an optimal distance for SERS enhancement. The generation of a measurable signal of the Raman spectrum is by elicitation of surface-enhanced plasmon resonance by laser excitation. The analytical sensitivity is of nano molar range.

5. *Diagnosis by restriction fragment length polymorphisms and related DNA-based approaches-* The RFLP is based on variation in genome sequences even in closely related organisms. RFLPs have a clear value for use in epidemiological studies. The use of pulsed-field gel electrophoresis (PFGE) results in the separation of large fragments of DNA and can be a very useful tool in addition to RFLP analysis. Random amplified polymorphic DNA (RAPD) is performed using 8–12-mer random primers that will or will not amplify a segment of DNA based on complementarity to the primers' sequence. Although the RFLP and PCR-RFLP are much less useful compared with the recent sequencing technologies, they are less expensive, easy to carry out and sufficiently descriptive for epidemiological investigations

6. *Genome sequencing* Compared with conventional targeted sequencing, high-throughput sequencing have shown much greater diagnostic opportunities, Next-generation sequencing (NGS) allows the sequencing of a large genome in a short time, facilitating the study of genetic material (DNA/RNA) recovered directly from clinical and environmental samples.

7. *Diagnosis by DNA probes and DNA microarray technology* Probes are known short nucleic acids which can hybridize with the target nucleic acid. Labeled probes help in detection after hybridization. Hybridization may be carried out in solution or solid phase or also in-situ.

Reverse line blotting has been used for diagnosis of theileriosis and babesiosis. PCR-ELISA is reported to be at least 1000 times more sensitive than thin blood smears for detection of *B. bovis*.

In Microarray technology, specific oligonucleotides are bound to small solid supports such as glass slides, silicon chips or nylon membranes. Extracted DNA or complementary DNA is labeled with a fluorescent dye and then hybridized with the microarray. Specific patterns of fluorescence are detected by a microarray reader which allows the identification of specific gene sequences found only in the pathogen of interest.

Nanotechnology

The term 'nanotechnology' is broadly defined as systems or devices related to the features of nanometre scale. One advantage of this technology is the potential to analyse a sample for an array of infectious agents on a single chip. Nano particle technology include the use of gold nanoparticles, nanobarcodes, quantum dots (cadmium selenide) and nanoparticle probes to label antibodies which can be used in various assays to identify specific pathogens.

Novel Biotechnological Tools in Control

Recombinant Vaccines

Molecular techniques can be used to produce a variety of different constructs of haemoprotozoal agents, and offer several advantages over conventional vaccines such as the deletion of the virulent gene(s) responsible for the disease, increased stability (which is an advantage for their effective use in developing countries), differentiation between infected and vaccinated animals through detecting antibodies either against unique proteins in the vaccine or not detecting antibodies against the deleted gene/protein (DIVA vaccines).

Sterile Insect Technique (SIT)

Virgin female insects are allowed to mate with sterile male insects and they do not produce any offspring. Repeated releases of mass-produced sterile insects help in containing, controlling or eradicating the insects. SIT is an important component of insect management for controlling the tsetse and in turn trypanosomiasis disease burden in some countries.

The most important applications of biotechnology for sensitive and specific diagnostic techniques and improved vaccines with efficient delivery systems in animal health may improve animal disease control significantly, thereby promoting both food production and livestock trade.

Further Readings

1. Schmitt B and Henderson L. (2005). Diagnostic tools for animal diseases. *Rev. sci. tech. Off. int. Epiz.*, 24(1), 243-250.

2. Biotechnology in the diagnosis of infectious diseases Version adopted by the World Assembly of Delegates of the OIE in May (2012). http://www.oie.int/fileadmin/Home/eng/Health_standards/tahm/GUIDE_3.2_BIOTECH_DIAG_INF_DIS.pdf

3. Gubbels J M., De Vos A P, Van Der Weide M, Viseras J, Schouls L. M, De Vries E and Jongejan F (1999). Simultaneous detection of bovine *Theileria* and *Babesia* species by reverse line blot hybridization. *J Clin Microbiol.* 37(6), 1782–1789.

Chapter 12

Sampling Techniques and Herd Level Sample Size Estimation

K.P. Suresh and M.R. Gajendragad

*ICAR-National Institute of Veterinary Epidemiology and
Disease Informatics (NIVEDI), Post Box No. 6450,
Ramagondanahalli, Yelahanka, Bengaluru – 560 064, Karnataka*

Sampling Techniques

Epidemiological studies usually involve sampling from livestock populations in some way in order to make inferences about a disease or diseases present in these populations. The units sampled are referred to as *sample units*. Sample units may be individual animals or they may be the units that contain the. animals to be investigated, such as herd, ranch, farm, or village. The *sample fraction* is the number of units actually sampled, divided by the total number of units in the population being sampled. A population can be defined as including all animals or items with the features one wishes to understand, because there is very rarely enough time or money to gather information from everyone or everything in a population, the goal becomes finding a representative sample of that population.

Sampling may be defined as the selection of some part of an aggregate or totality on the basis of which a judgement or inference about the aggregate or totality is made. In other words it is the process of obtaining information about an entire population by examining only a part of it. In most of the research work and surveys the usual approach happens to be make generalization or to draw inferences based on samples about the parameters of population from which the population are taken.

Sampling is used in practice for a variety of reasons such as:

i) Sampling is cheaper than census method. It is economical too.

ii) As the magnitude of operations is small in case of sampling, so data collection and analysis can be carried out accurately and efficiently.

iii) Sampling is the only way when the population is as large as the population of a country.

iv) Sampling enables the researcher to make a precise estimate of the standard error which helps in obtaining information concerning some characteristic of the population

Sampling Frame

A sampling frame can be defined as the list consisting of the units of the population. One very necessary and critical point to be kept in mind in case of the sampling frame is that it should be made up to date and also it should be free from the various errors of the omission and duplication of the sampling units. In many cases, it has been observed that the preparation of the sampling frame sometimes becomes a very critical practical problem.

A perfect frame is the one that is able to identify each element only once and these frames are very rarely available in the real life. A sampling frame may consist of different types of defects and these defects can be classified on the following lines

(1) Incomplete frame: some legitimate sampling units of population are omitted

(2) Inaccurate frame: some of the sampling units are inaccurately listed or sometimes such units are involved which actually are not existing.

(3) Inadequate frame: Does not include all the units of the population by its structure.

Area Frame

An area frame, a set of geographical areas, is always complete, and remains useful a long time. The completeness of area frames suggests their use in many cases, for example: a) if other complete frame is not available; b) if an existing list of sampling units change very rapidly; c) if an existing frame is out of date; d) if an existing frame was obtained from a census with a low coverage; e) if a multiple purpose frame is needed for estimating many different variables (agricultural, environmental, livestock disease *etc.*).

Area frame sample designs allow objective estimates of characteristics of interest (livestock disease) that can be observed on the ground, without interviews; besides, the materials used for the survey and the information collected help to reduce non sampling errors in interviews and are a good basis for data imputation for non-respondents; finally, the area sample survey materials are becoming cheaper and more accurate.

Area frame sample designs also have some disadvantages, such as the cost of implementing the survey program, the necessity of more cartographic materials, the sensitivity to outliers and the instability of estimates. If the survey is conducted through interviews and respondents live far from the selected area unit, their identification may be difficult and expensive, and missing data tend to be relevant.

Sampling methods are broadly categorized into two groups:

A. Probability Sampling Methods
- ☆ Simple random sampling
- ☆ Stratified random sampling
- ☆ Systematic random sampling
- ☆ Cluster random sampling
- ☆ Adaptive cluster sampling
- ☆ Multistage sampling
- ☆ Area sampling

B. Non-Probability Sampling Methods
- ☆ Convenience sampling
- ☆ Purposive sampling
- ☆ Quota sampling

Herd and Animal Level Sample Size Estimation

In a large population where animals are separated into herds, disease has a strong tendency to cluster. This is because the disease agent or agents (whether infectious, environmental or genetic) are generally not evenly distributed throughout the population (Rothman, 1990). With rare diseases, this clustering is usually even more pronounced. As a result, a very low proportion of herds may be affected by a particular disease-but within those affected herds, the prevalence of the disease amongst animals may be quite high. If a survey designed to detect the presence of disease fails to take into account the clustering of disease in the population, the results of the survey are likely to be very unreliable. This is because the probability formulae that the surveys are based on assume that every unit in the population has the same probability of being affected. Another problem with large-area surveys is the logistics of sampling. Probability formulae assume simple random sampling. Simple random sampling of individual animals from a national herd requires the creation of a sampling frame which may need to list millions of animals (each uniquely identified). Such a sampling frame is usually impossible to construct.

The solution to both these problems is to use a two-stage sampling strategy in which herds form the first stage, and individual animals within selected herds, the second stage. In this way, the sample sizes at each stage can be adjusted to reflect the different disease prevalences (the proportion of herds affected in the first stage, and the proportion of animals affected in the herd at the second stage). Two-stage sampling also means that the construction of sampling frames is much simpler. At the first stage, only a list of all herds in the population is required, and at the second stage, only animals in each of the selected herds is to be included in the list. However, the use of two-stage sampling presents particular problems for sample-size calculation and analysis.

The use of two-stage sampling has evolved to meet surveillance objectives for two reasons. First, list of frames of animals for randomized sample selection do not typically exist at a regional or national level, but the list frames of herds can be developed and maintained more readily. Secondly, the theory and applications of within-herd sampling with imperfect diagnostic tests is well developed. The within-herd sampling research has guided the approach to sampling to classify the herd's disease or infection status.

The herd-level sensitivity (HSe or HSESNS) and Specificity (HSp or HSEPC) depend on the individual animal test characteristics, sample size, within herd prevalence *etc.*, HSe and HSp are test characteristics which can be applied at the herd level in a manner equivalent to animal-level Sensitivity (Se) and Specificity(Sp) at the within -herd level. HSe and HSp usually are based on detecting infection if it is present above a fixed level, that is the level is determined according to the epidemiology of the disease or specific national or international rules.

Further Readings

1. Cannon, R.M., (2001). Sense and sensitivity – designing surveys based on an imperfect test. *Prev. Vet. Med.* 49, 141–163.

2. Cannon, R.M., Roe, R.T., (1982). Livestock Disease Surveys – A Field Manual for Veterinarians. Canberra.

3. Collins, M.T., Sockett, D.C., Goodger, W.J., Conrad, T.A., Thomas, C.B., Carr, D.J., (1994). Herd prevalence and geographic-distribution of, and risk- factors for, bovine paratuberculosis in Wisconsin. *J. Am. Vet. Med. Assoc.* 204, 636–641.

4. Snedecor, G.W., Cochrane,W.G., (1989). Statistical Methods, 6th ed. Iowa State University Press, Ames, Iowa, p.121.

5. Lemeshow S, Stroh G Jr., (1998). Sampling Techniques for Evaluating Health Parameters in Developing Countries. National Academy Press, Washington D.C.

6. Schaeffer RL, Mendenhall W, Ott L., (1990). Elementary Survey Sampling, Fourth Edition. Duxbury Press, Belmont, California.

Chapter 13

Estimation of Socio-Economic Losses Due to Animal Diseases

G. Govindaraj and P. Krishnamoorthy

ICAR-National Institute of Veterinary Epidemiology and Disease Informatics (NIVEDI), Post Box No. 6450, Ramagondanahalli, Yelahanka, Bengaluru – 560 064, Karnataka

The effect of disease in animals reduces the efficiency with which inputs are converted into outputs. Besides this there are several direct and indirect effects of which some can be valued or quantified easily and some are difficult to quantify. Besides quantification using the reliable data collected from primary or secondary sources, the effect of a disease can be modeled by implying certain assumptions like increased death rate, lower yield, decreased body weight, increased calving/ kidding interval *etc.* It is also sometimes referred as simulation assessment of the impact of the disease.

Disease Impact

Any disease in animals has direct and indirect impacts on the performance of animals and on animal keepers. The direct impact can be further classified into visible and invisible impacts. The visible impacts can be easily quantified. *e.g.* mortality loss, reduction in milk, wool reduction in draught power, money expended on vaccines and veterinarians fee. The invisible impacts due to a disease are reduced fertility and changed herd structure. The quantification of invisible losses can be made using certain models and assumptions since the exact information/data is not usually available and are difficult to obtain.

The indirect impact includes societal and financial impact. The non-disposal of dead animals in the scientific manner has impact on environment through release of harmful gases or spread of disease to disease free herds/animals in the neighborhood. The death of animals in large numbers in general or death of certain breeds/species due to outbreaks in a certain geographical region has variable societal impact. The indirect impact like change in methane gas emission levels, change in dung availability and its impact on agriculture and allied activities productivity, change in carrying capacity *etc.*, also affects the society at large due to disease in animals. The death of animal also affects the availability of animal products like milk to the farm family especially in subsistence agriculture families. It also affects the human nutrition and thereby reduces the longevity. It also ends up in various social problems in the long run. The indirect impact of zoonotic diseases affects humans and has larger societal ramifications.

The indirect financial impact includes lesser price for the diseased animals in the market or lower value for the normal animals also in a particular locality due to an outbreak. The price of the complement and substitute goods also changes due a disease outbreak and hence the price effect should be a part of impact analysis.

All the above impacts have to be quantified in a scientific manner so as to arrive the overall impact of the disease. Quantifying the direct impact of any disease is relatively easy compared to quantifying the indirect impact. However, with use of implicit assumptions and indirect valuation methods the overall impact can be quantified.

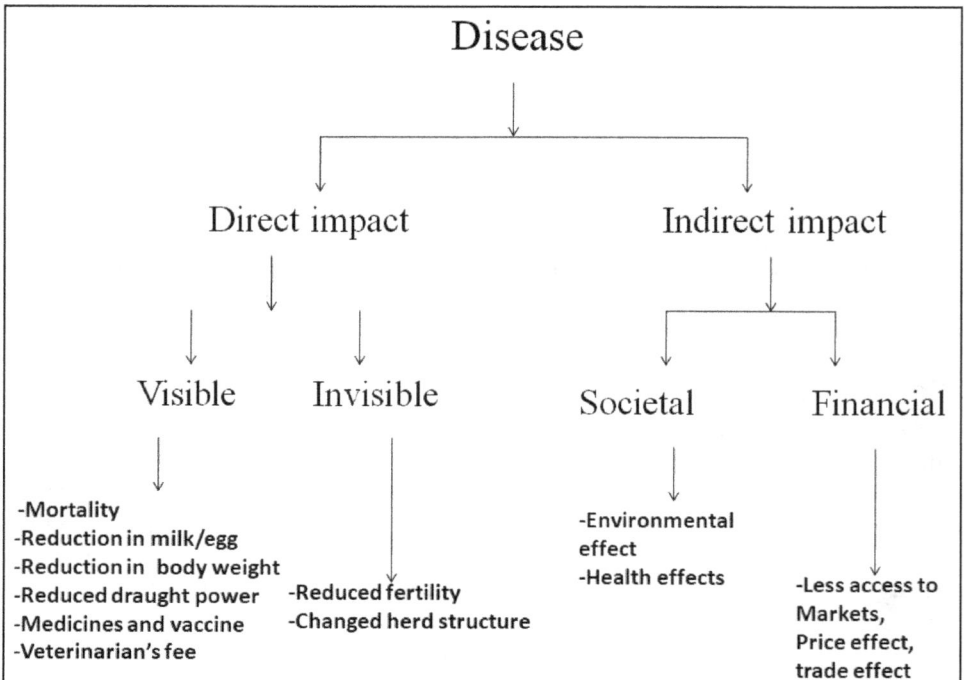

Information Required for Developing a Disease Economic Module

i) The foremost information required is about the disease itself, *i.e.*

    a) whether the disease is bacterial or viral or parasitic or combination thereof or any other agent?

    b) incidence rate of the disease

    c) duration of infection

ii) Diseased animal information

    a) The species information (*E.g.* bovine, small ruminants, poultry, pig, horse, *etc.*)

    b) The breed details (*E.g.* indigenous, crossbred, exotic)

    c) The age and sex of the diseased animal

    d) The susceptibility information agewise, sexwise, breedwise

iii The physiological parameters at normal and diseased state

iv) Productive and economic traits at normal and diseased state

Indicators Required for Assessing the Losses

The indicators required for assessing the losses due to animal diseases may vary for macro (national) or micro (farm) level estimation. The important indicators required for macro level disease impact estimates are as follows:

a) The number of animals died in different species and across different ages

b) The number of animals culled due to disease in different species and across different ages

c) The number of animals disabled due to disease in different species and across different ages

d) The productivity loss in animals like milk loss/day/animal

e) The number of days of milking loss in a lactation *etc.*

f) The number of days of draught power loss due to a disease

g) Information on decreased levels of fertility

h) Information on incidence of abortion

i) Changes in herd structure due to a disease

j) Loss due to non- access to markets

k) Treatment cost on drugs and vaccines

l) The cost of manpower/labour

Besides, the basic requirements listed above the economic information are also necessary to assess the impact of the disease. For time series disease impact assessment, the data on different time periods are necessary whereas for the cross section analysis the information during a particular time on different variables are required.

Some of the very important economic information required are given below:

a) Price of milk, wool, meat, *etc.*

b) Price of live animal for different breeds, for different age groups and for different sex

c) Price of the culled animal for different breeds, for different age groups and for different sex

d) Price of disabled animal across breeds, age and sex

e) Rates of bullock labour per day

f) Rates of hired labour per day for male and female

g) Own price variation and change in prices of complements and substitutes

h) Veterinarian or para-veterinarians fee

The information listed above is necessary to assess the losses due to a disease. However, depending on the disease and level of the study the data requirements vary.

Loss Assessment Types

A) Cross Sectional Loss Analysis

The loss due to a disease is assessed based on the data collected at a particular time point across the stake holders.

Advantages

a) The estimates are authentic provided the time of data collection, sample size, sampling methods *etc.*, followed are appropriate.

b) Does not rely on other sources of information.

Disadvantages

a) The estimates represent the assessment period only.

b) Cost and time involved are high.

c) The estimates would be inconsistent, if appropriate sampling procedures are not followed.

B) With and Without

This method can be used for quantifying the changes in losses due to an intervention or policy action. For example, Government of India had initiated PPR control programmes in sheep and goat during 2010-11 and the benefits or loss minimization due to this intervention can be assessed by with and without method.

C) Before and After

This method can be used for assessing the losses before and after the outbreak of a disease. For example, our country is now free from Rinderpest due to the successful implementation of control programme for this disease. The benefits/ impact of such programme can be assessed by following this approach.

Models to Assess the Direct and Indirect Losses

The disease loss module comprises several models for quantifying the loss. The models depend on the type of animal affected, extent of direct loss due to a disease like mortality, milk reduction, reduction in body weight, reduction in draught power etc and on the extent of indirect impact like health effect, environmental effect and price effect. The examples of models for assessing the loss due to PPR in sheep and goat are presented below:

Losses due to Mortality

$$M = D \times P$$

where,

M = Loss due to mortality'
D = Number of animals died
P = Price of the animal in that particular year

Loss due to Reduction in Milk Yield (examples)

a) *Direct loss due reduction in milk yield*

$$DM = (I-D) \, P_r \, P_l \, M_y \, P_m$$

where,

DM = Direct Milk Loss (Rs)
I = Incidence
D = Deaths
P_r = Proportion of animals in milk
P_l = Proportion of lactation lost(per cent)
M_y = Milk yield per milch animal
P_m = Price of milk in respective year(Rs/kg)

b) *Milk loss due to increased inter-kidding period*

$$MIK = [(12/K) - \{12/(K+W)\}] \, (I-D) \, P_r \, Y \, P_m$$

where,

MIK = Milk loss due to increase in inter-kidding period
K = Inter kidding period (months)
W = Delay in next conception (months)
I = Incidence
D = Deaths
P_r = Proportion of animals in milk

Y = Annual average milk yield per animal in milk

P_m = Price of milk of respective years (Rs/kg)

c) Milk loss due to increased abortions

$$MA= [(12/K)-\{12/(K+9.5\ A)\}]\ (I-D)\ P_r\ Y\ P_m$$

where,

MA = Milk loss due to increased abortions

K = Inter kidding period (months)

A = increased abortion rate (per cent)

I = Incidence

D = Deaths

P_r = Proportion of animals in milk(per cent)

Y = Annual average milk yield per animal in milk

P_m = Price of milk in respective year (Rs/kg)

The increased abortion leads to prolonged inter-kidding period besides loss of kids. Assuming the time for abortion as 3.5 months from conception, and a delay of six months in the next conception, inter- kidding would be increased by 9.5 months.

Conclusions

The economic losses due to diseases in livestock are broadly put into two main classes, *viz.,* mortality losses and morbidity losses. The mortality losses include the value loss due to death of an adult animal and the value loss of calves due to mortality and abortion. The morbidity losses can be grouped into four major classes, *viz.,* production loss, reproductive loss, treatment costs and miscellaneous costs. The data on the various physical and economic aspects mentioned are necessary to estimate the economic losses due to diseases in livestock.

The analysis of disease losses from different angles helps the farmers as well as policy makers and planners. The estimation of losses species-wise tells farmers which species are more susceptible to diseases and by how much and thus they can manage to reduce losses in livestock. Similarly, age or herd size-wise estimate of losses suggest them at what age the animal is more susceptible. An analysis of losses due to many diseases at a time indicates which diseases are more deadly or damaging so that they can be managed accordingly. The disease loss information also help policy makers and planners to decide which disease ranks first in terms of losses so that they can get due importance in policy planning. It is also useful for persons dealing with livestock insurance in terms of deciding premiums for different species, age groups and size of animals.

Chapter 14

Identification, Isolation and Maintenance of *Trypanosoma evansi* *In vitro* and *In vivo*

P.P. Sengupta and M. Ligi

ICAR-National Institute of Veterinary Epidemiology and Disease Informatics (NIVEDI), Post Box No. 6450, Ramagondanahalli, Yelahanka, Bengaluru – 560 064, Karnataka

In all Haemoprotozoan diseases preparation of appropriate blood smear preparation is at most necessary. A perfect blood smear can reveal not only parasites but also the physiological condition of the animal. Romanowsky's blood smear staining procedure is very useful.

Revival of *T. evansi* Stabilates

a) Different isolates of *T.evansi* isolates (buffalo, dog, lion and leopard) are maintained in our laboratory, *in-vitro* in liquid nitrogen.

b) The stabilates maintained in the laboratory (*in-vitro*) are revived by infecting into rats/mice.

c) For infecting the rat, the vials taken from the LN_2 are thawed immediately and blood from capillary tubes is transferred to small beakers.

d) Depending upon the number of rats/mice, blood is equally distributed and administered intraperitoneally/intradermally using 1ml disposable syringe

Screening of Infected Animal

1. Parasite level in rat/mice can be checked by collecting the blood (10-20µl) from the tail end.

2. Wipe tail end of the animal with 70 per cent alcohol and pierce a sterile needle.

3. Draw the blood on to a glass slide and make a clear smear

4. Allow the smear to dry and fix it by methanol for 1 minute

5. Add Geimsa stain (1:4 diluted) (1ml of stain +8ml of phosphate buffer) and allow it for 45min.

6. Wash it with tap water and allow it to dry

7. Observe under the microscope (100X) for the presence of parasite.

8. At very high parasitaemia (usually 30-40 tryps/field) sacrifice the animal and collect the blood from the heart with 2 per cent EDTA.

Dissection

Materials Required

Disposable syringe (5ml), 2 per cent EDTA as anticoagulant, normal Saline, beakers with EDTA, chloroform and dessicator, glass slides (grease free)

Procedure

1. Euthanize the infected animal and transfer to the dissecting tray

2. Dissect the animal and cut open the chest muscle to draw blood from the heart

3. Rinse 5 ml disposable syringe with 2 per cent EDTA and draw blood from the heart.

4. Transfer the collected blood to the glass beakers slowly containing 2 per cent EDTA.

5. Continuously and slowly stir the beaker to avoid clotting of blood.

6. Once the entire blood is collected from the heart, separate the plasma/ buffy coat to purify the trypanosomes.

Purification of Trypanosomes

Trypanosomes from the blood/plasma can be purified by diethylaminoethyl (DEAE) anion-exchange column chromatography.

Equilibration of DEAE-cellulose

1. Suspend fifty gram of DEAE-cellulose in 2 liters of distilled water and mix for 20 minutes with a magnetic stirrer at low speed.

2. Adjust the pH to 8 with ortho-phosphoric acid and allow to settle for 30 minutes.

3. Discard the supernatant fluid containing the finest granules and repeat the procedure three times.

4. Store the equilibrated, concentrated slurry (DEAE-cellulose) in small aliquots at –20°C for till further use.

Packing of the Column with Equilibrated DEAE-Cellulose

1. For packing of chromatographic glass column (10 ml), place a disc of Whatman No. 41 filter paper at the bottom of the syringe (column) and moisten by adding a few drops of PSG.

2. Fit the column to burette stand and add equilibrated cellulose slurry (~4 ml) into the syringe and allow packing for few minutes before elution of the buffer.

3. Wash the column later and equilibrate with 2 ml of PSG without disturbing the surface (the height of the sediment can be approximately 3cm).

Adsorption of Trypanosomes

1. Centrifuge the heparinized blood at 3000 rpm for 3 minutes to collect the buffy coat.

2. Add the buffy coat on to the surface of the cellulose column and allow it penetrate the cellulose. The cellulose column was kept moistened throughout the procedure.

3. Add PSG (~2 ml) on to the column to elute the trypanosomes.

4. Collect the elution in 15 ml centrifuge tube and centrifuge at 1000g for 10 minutes.

5. Observe the elution under the microscope by placing a drop of elute on the glass slide for trypanosomes.

Chapter 15

Diagnosis of Parasite by PCR Technique

M. Ligi and P.P. Sengupta

ICAR-National Institute of Veterinary Epidemiology and
Disease Informatics (NIVEDI), Post Box No. 6450,
Ramagondanahalli, Yelahanka, Bengaluru – 560 064, Karnataka

Introduction

The polymerase chain reaction (PCR) is the cardinal laboratory technology of molecular biology. It is one of the most powerful laboratory techniques ever discovered. PCR combines the unique attributes of being very sensitive and specific with a great degree of flexibility. With the PCR it is possible to specifically address a particular DNA sequence and to amplify this sequence to extremely high copy numbers. Since its initial development in the early 1980's, dozens of variations in the basic theme of PCR have successfully been carried out. In fact, the very flexibility and application-specific variation of PCR make it seem like there are as many ways to do a PCR reactions there are researchers doing them. Here, a basic, straight-forward PCR protocol is presented. Where appropriate, some of the choices for modifying this standard reaction that are routinely available to researchers are discussed.

Step 1: Choosing Target Substrates and PCR Primers

The choice of the target DNA is, of course, dictated by the specific experiment. However, one thing is common to all substrate DNAs and that is they must be as clean a possible and uncontaminated with other DNAs. Naturally, if the source material is an environmental sample such as water or soil, then the researcher must rely upon the specificity of the PCR primers to avoid amplification of the wrong thing. Specificity in the choice of PCR primers should be an issue in any PCR amplification.

The on-line IDT SciTools software OligoAnalyzer 3.0 and PrimerQuest are invaluable aids both in primer design and validation. PrimerQuest will assist in primer design and will permit the researcher to directly assess primer specificity via a direct BLAST search of the candidate sequences.Taking candidate primer sequences into OligoAnalyzer will allow for each primer sequence to be assessed for the presence of secondary structures whether these are hairpins or homo- and hetero-dimers.

Step 2: Setting Up the Reaction

Once you have chosen the appropriate substrate and your PCR primer sequences and you have them on hand, the basic reaction components are as follows:

1. Nuclease free water
2. 10x Reaction Buffer
3. $MgCl_2$
4. dNTPs
5. Forward Primer
5. Reverse Primer
7. Target DNA
8. Polymerase enzyme

One common choice available to the researcher is whether or not to use a Reaction Buffer that already contains the magnesium chloride. The vast majority of PCR reactions will work perfectly well at a 1.5 millimolar (mM) magnesium chloride concentration. For this reason PCR reaction buffers that do contain MgCl2 are prepared so that the final concentration is 1.5mM in the 1:10 dilution. Occasionally, however, MgCl2 final concentrations other than 1.5mM may be optimal.When this occurs it becomes necessary to use a reaction buffer that does not contain MgCl2 and to add the MgCl2 separately.

Step 3: Choosing the Reaction Conditions

The reaction conditions of PCR amplification are composed of the total number of cycles to be run and the temperature and duration of each step in those cycles. The decision as to how many cycles to run is based upon the amount of DNA target material you start with as well as how many copies of the PCR product (amplicon) you want. In general, 25 to 35 cycles is the standard for a PCR reaction. This results in from approximately 34 million to 34 billion copies of the desired sequence using 25 cycles and 35 cycles respectively. Additional cycle numbers can be used if there is a small amount of target DNA available for the reaction. However, reactions in excess of 45 cycles are quite rare. Also, increasing the number of cycles for larger amounts of starting material is counterproductive because the presence of very high concentrations of the PCR product is itself inhibitory (see Kainz, 2000).

Once the number of cycles is selected, it is necessary to choose the temperature and duration of each step in the cycles. The first step is the DNA denaturation step that renders the entire DNA in the reaction single stranded. This is routinely accomplished at 94oC or 95oC for 30 seconds. The second step is the primer annealing step during which the PCR primers find their complementary targets and attach themselves to those sequences. Here the choice of temperature is largely determined by the melting temperature (Tm) of the two PCR primers (see OligoAnalyzer 3.0 in IDT SciTools). Again, the usual duration is 30 seconds. Finally, the last step in a PCR cycle is the polymerase extension step during which the DNA polymerase is producing a complimentary copy of the target DNA strand starting from the PCR primer sequence (thus the term primer). The usual temperature of this step is 72 °C, considered to be a good optimum temperature for thermal-stable polymerases. A common rule of thumb for the duration of this step has been 30 seconds for every 500 bases in the PCR product. However, with the increasing quality of commercially available polymerase enzymes and the associated reaction components, this time can be significantly shortened but should be done in a systematic manner since the optimal extension time can be polymerase and sequence specific. In addition to these cycling conditions, it is often desirable to place a single denaturation step of three to five minutes at 94°C or 95°C at the beginning of the reaction and a final extension step of a few minutes at 72°C. A convenient shorthand way of representing a complete set of reaction conditions is: initial denaturation at 94°C for 5 min, followed by 35 cycles of denaturation at 94°C for 1 min, annealing at 600C for 45 sec, primer extension at 72°C for 2 min, and final extension at 720C for 10 min.

Step 4: Validating the Reaction

Once your PCR reaction has run, there are two ways of determining success or failure. The first is to simply take some of the final reaction and run it out on an agarose gel with an appropriate molecular weight marker to make sure that the reaction was successful and if the amplified product is the expected size relative to the maker.The ultimate validation of a PCR reaction is to directly sequence the amplicon.

For carrying out PCR from any sample, first DNA has to be isolated and confirmed.

Below are few methods for DNA isolation from different sources:

BLOOD AND BODY FLUID SPIN PROTOCOL (Protocol is followed from QIAGEN QIAamp® DNA Mini kit handbook)

Note

☆ Equilibrate samples to room temperature (15°C-25°C)

☆ Heat a water bath or heating block at 56c

☆ Keep ready buffer AL, buffer AW1, Buffer AW2, QIAGEN Protease from the kit

☆ All centrifugation steps should be carried out at room temperature

☆ 200µl of whole blood yields 3-12 µg of DNA

Protocol

☆ Pipette 20µl QIAGEN protease (or Proteinase K) into the bottom of a 1.5 ml micro centrifuge tube.

☆ Add 200µl sample to the micro centrifuge tube (Blood samples)

Note: It is possible to add QIAGEN protease (or proteinase K) to the samples that have already been dispensed into microcentrifuge tubes. In this case, it is important to ensure proper mixing after adding the enzyme

☆ Add 200µl Buffer AL to the sample. Mix by pulse vortexing for 15s. (In order to ensure efficient lysis, it is essential that the sample and buffer AL are mixed thoroughly to yield a homogeneous solution. (Note: Do not add QIAGEN Protease or Proteinase K directly to Buffer AL)

☆ Incubate at 56°C for 10 minutes in water bath or heating block

☆ (DNA yield reached a maximum after lysis for 10 minutes at 56°C)

☆ Briefly centrifuge the 1.5 ml micro centrifuge tube to remove drops from the inside the lid.

☆ Add 200µl ethanol (96-100 per cent) to the sample, and mix again by pulse- vortexing for 15 s. After mixing briefly centrifuge the 1.5 ml micro centrifuge tube to remove drops from the inside the lid.

☆ Carefully apply the mixture from the step 6 to the QIAamp spin Column (in a 20 ml collection tube) without wetting the rim, close the cap, and centrifuge at 8000 rpm, for 1 minutes. Place the QIAamp spin Coloum in a clean 2 ml collection tube (provided) and discard the tube containing the filterate.

☆ Carefully open the QIAamp spin Column and add 500µl buffer AWI without wetting the rim. Close the cap and centrifuge at 8000rpm for 1 mints Place the QIAamp spin Column in a clean 2ml collection tube (Provided) and discard the collection tube containing filter ate

☆ Carefully open the QIAamp spin Column and add 500µl buffer AW2 without wetting the rim close the cap and centrifuge at full (14000rmp) for 5 mint

☆ Place the QIAamp spin Column in a new 2ml collection tube and discard the collection tube with the filterate. Centrifuge at 14000rpm for 2mints

☆ Place the QIAamp spin Column in a clean 1.5ml micro centrifuge tube and discard the collection tube containing the filter rate

☆ Place the QIAamp spin Column in a clean 1.5 ml micro centrifuge tube and discard the collection tube containing the filter ate.carefully open the QIAamp spin Column and add 50µl buffer AE

☆ In cubate at room temperature for 5 minutes and then centrifuge at 8000rpm for 2 minutes (this is first elution)

☆ 2nd elution step with a further 200µl buffer AE will increase yield by up to 15 per cent (Repeat the same procedure as above)

☆ DNA containing elution solution is preserved at -80°c

DNA ISOLATION FROM TISSUE FROM QIAamp DNA MINI KIT ONLY (Usually snail tissue)

Protocol

☆ Cut up to 25mg tissue into small pieces

☆ Place in a 1.5ml micro centrifuge tube (Round bottom is preferred)

☆ Add 180μl of buffer ATL

☆ Add 20 μl proteinase K, and mix by vortexing

☆ Keep it for incubation at 56 c for 1 hrs in water bath until the tissue is completely lysed

☆ Centrifuge (short spin) to remove drops from the inside of the lid

☆ Add 200 μl buffer AL to the sample, mix by pulse-vortexing for 15sec and incubate at 70c for 10 mints. Briefly centrifuge the 1.5ml centrifuge tube to remove drops from inside the lid. (In water bath)

☆ Add 200μl ethanol (96-100 per cent)

☆ Mix by vortexing for 15 sec

☆ Briefly centrifuge to remove drops from inside the lid

☆ Transfer the above mixture to the collection tube through spin Column without wetting the rim (lid)

☆ Close the cap and centrifuge at 6000rpm for 1 mints

☆ Place the QIAamp spin Column in a clean 2 ml collection tube (provided) and discard the tube containing the filterate.

☆ Carefully open the QIAamp spin Column and add 500μl buffer AW1 without wetting the rim.

☆ Close the cap and centrifuge at 6000 rpm for 1 minutes

☆ Place the QIAamp spin Column in a clean 2 ml collection tube (provided) and discard the collection tube containing the filter ate.

☆ Carefully open the QIAamp spin Column and add 500μl buffer AW2 without wetting the rim

☆ Close the cap and centrifuge at full speed (*i.e.* 14000 rpm) for 3 minutes

☆ Replace the spin Column in a clean (new) 1.5μl microcentrifuge tube and discard the old collection tube containing filterate

☆ Open the spin Column and add 50μl of buffer AE or dH20

☆ Incubate at room temperature for 5 minutes

☆ Centrifuge a 6000 rpm for 1 minutes

☆ Collect the DNA eluted and label as E1 and store at -20°C

Once the DNA sample is ready for PCR, carry out PCR by using appropriate primer

Diagnostic primers developed for detection of trypanosomiasis in our laboratory

PCR Based Diagnosis Exploring VSG

Two pairs of primers - DITRYF/R and EXP3F/4R were designed in our laboratory from the published sequences, respectively from accession number EF495337 and AF317924 available in the GenBank data base. The PCR primer pair DITRYF/R was used to amplify the genomic DNA (400bp), while EXP3F/4R was used to amplify (1432bp) the cDNA synthesized from VSG mRNA.

DITRY F/R

Primer set targeting variable surface glycoprotein (VSG) of *T.evansi*

GenBank No: E7495337 (VSG gene of *T. evansi*)

DITRY F- **5'- CGA CCA GCC AGA ACG AGC AGA AT- 3'** (23 mer)

(Corresponding to 721-743 bp)

DITRY R-**5'- CTT GTC GAT CGA GTT GAC GGT- 3'**) (21 mer)

(Corresponding to 1090-1111bp)

PCR Reaction

☆ Initial Denaturation- 94°C- 3min

☆ Denaturation- 94°C, 1-min (35 cycles)

☆ Primer annealing-54°C- 1min

☆ Primer Extension-72°C- 10min

TeDISGF/R

Primer set targeting invariable surface glycoprotein (ISG) of *T.evansi*

GenBank accession no. - JN797772

TeD-ISGF (5' CAG CCG GTG AGT GAA GAA A 3') (Corresponding to 1072-1090bp)

TeD-ISGR (5' CTA CGG CCC CTA ATA ATA AAG AAC 3') (Corresponding to 1478-1455bp)

PCR Reaction

☆ Initial denaturation- 3min at 98°C

☆ Denaturation-30 sec at 98°C

☆ Primer annealing- 1min at 53°C

☆ Primer extension- 1min at 72°C

☆ Final primer extension-10 m at 72°C

☆ **Primers used for detection of fasciola in snail tissue is FASSNAIL and ITS-2**

Preparation of 50μl PCR Reaction Mixture

Add,

NFW	32.5μl
Taq buffer	5μl
Mgcl2(50mM)	4μl
dNTPs (10mM)	1 μl
Primer A	1 μl
Primer B	1μl
Taq DNA Polymerase	0.5 μl (3 units)
DNA	5μl

Protocol for PCR

☆ Add all the above ingredient into PCR tubes (50μl reaction mixture)

☆ Prepare one PCR tube with positive control (known DNA) and another tube with negative control (with out DNA)

☆ Keep all the tubes in thermo cycler (PCR machine)

☆ Set the programme of the primer

☆ Run the programme

☆ Take out the PCR tubes from PCR machine

☆ Load the mixture in the gel

☆ Observe the band

Checking the Band through Gel Electrophoresis

Usually we prepare 1 per cent agarose gel

Preparation

0.5 gm Agarose +15ml 1X TAE + 35ml dH20 (For small Gel preparation)

1 gm Agarose + 30 ml 1X TAE + 70 ml d H2O (For big Gel preparation)

Protocol

☆ Keep the gel electrophoresis apparatus ready

☆ Mix 1 gm Agarose + 30ml 1XTAE + 70 ml dH2O (for bigger Gel)

☆ Heat the mix in microwave oven for 30 sec (3 times) for proper melting of Agar

☆ Cool the Mixture by showing it through running tap water or placing it in water bath

☆ After cooling add 5-6 μl of EtBr to the mixture and mix it

(Note: Always use Gloves while handling EtBr)

☆ Pour the mixture electrophoresis apparatus (cascade)

☆ Allow it to solidify

☆ Once the gel is solidified, remove the comb carefully

☆ Add 0.5X TAE which is used as running buffer in the cascade (Note: Gel should be Completely submerged in the running buffer)

☆ For loading:

☆ Mix 5-10µl of DNA + 5µl of loading dye (we use orange dye), depending upon the capacity of the gel (20-50µl of mixture can be loaded in one big gel well)

☆ Once all the samples are loaded as mentioned above, connect the apparatus to the power pack

☆ Set the Volt to 60-80V. (Initially set it to 60V. Once the DNA band has reached half way, the volt can be increased to 100V

☆ Once all the bands have reached opposite sides, switch off the power pack and remove the gel carefully from the cascade (Note: Kindly wear gloves)

☆ Check the bands in Gel Documentation Machine (We use Biorad Gel Doc)

☆ Clear bands are visible and can be captured in the system which can be stored for future analysis.

Further Readings

1. Kainz, P (2000). The PCR plateau phase- towards an understanding of its limitations. Biochem Biophys Acta 1494: 23-27.There are a number of excellent resources for exploring the polymerase chain reaction and its variants. A few of these are listed below.

2. Bustin SA (2004). A to Z of Quantitative PCR. LaJolla, California: International Unniversity Line.

3. Chen B-Y, and HW Janes (2002). PCR Cloning Protocols, Second Edition. Totowa, New Jersey: Humana Press.

4. Dieffenbach CW, and GS Dveksler (2003). PCR Primer: A Laboratory Manual. Cold Spring Harbor, New York: Cold Spring Harbor Laboratory Press.

5. Harris E (1998). A Low-Cost Approach to PCR. Oxford: Oxford University Press.

6. Innis MA, DH Gelfand, JJ Sninsky, and TJ White (eds.) (1990). PCR Protocols: AGuide to Methods and Applications. San Diego, California: Academic Press.

8. McPherson MJ, SG Moller, R Beynon, and C Howe (2000). PCR: Basics from Background to Bench. Heidelberg: Springer-Verlag.

9. O'Connell J, and J O'Connell (2002). RT-PCR Protocols. Totowa, New Jersey: Humana Press.

0. Weissensteiner T, T Weissensteiner, HG Griffin, and AM Griffin (2003). PCR Technology: Current Innovations, Second Edition. Boca Raton, Florida: CRC Press.

Chapter 16

Identification of Different Arthropod Vectors Responsible for Haemoprotozoan Diseases and Determination of Insecticide Resistance

Placid E. D'Souza

CAFT in Veterinary Parasitology,
Veterinary College, KVAFSU, Hebbal, Bengaluru – 560 024, Karnataka

Tabanus spp.

Horse Fly/Breeze Fly/Gad Fly

These are very large flies with very large eyes and gap between them is small. Antennae are projected forward in front of the head and have 3 segments. The first 2 segments of the antenna are small, the third segment has 4 annulations and has a tooth like projection called spur. Flies hold their wings horizontally at rest. Proboscis is short The mouth part consists of two jointed well-developed palps, a pair of well developed mandibles and maxillae. Labrum epipharynx and hypopharynx are slender. Labium is well-developed with 2 prominent labella containing pseudotracheal tubes. When at rest, wings are not folded closely over the abdomen. Wings are strengthened with prominent veins and the third longitudinal vein is forked distally.

Chrysops spp.

Deer Fly

Mouth parts similar to that of *Tabanus* spp. Antenna is long and projected forward. All the 3 segments of antenna are elongate but the 3rd segment of antennae will not have a spur and has four annulations at its tip. Medium sized flies. Eyes are much smaller than *Tabanus* and the gap between them are large. Wings with a dark band across them and are held apart when at rest.

Haematopota spp.

Clegs

Size of these flies is intermediate between *Tabanus* and *Chrysops* Mouth parts are similar to *Tabanus* spp. Wings are held folded closed to abdomen and have a complex pattern of pigmentation. Wings have whitish blotches (mottled appearance) and at rest they meet at the base, diverge slightly and are held slightly sloping like the roof of a house. Eyes have zig zag bands. They have fairly large eyes with a wide gap between them. First segment of antennae is large, second is narrower and 3rd segment has 3 annulations. Spur is absent on the third segment. Antenna is projected forward.

Keys to Identify Ixodid Ticks of India

The Ixodid ticks otherwise known as hard ticks are so called because of the presence of a hard chitinous structure called scutum is present dorsally in all stages of life. The scutum covers the entire dorsum in case of male ticks and is restricted to the anterior region in larvae, nymphs and adult females. Articulations of the palps are varied. There are three prominent segments are generally present in palps and the fourth segment is reduced and it bears a chemoreceptor sensilla. Eyes if present are situated laterally on the scutum.

The females after engorging by sucking blood will fall off and lay eggs in crevices and holes in the floor of the animal shed. The eggs are small, round or oval in shape and brown in colour. From the eggs after the optimum incubation period larvae hatches out which are otherwise known as seed ticks which will have scutum and only three pairs of legs. These seed ticks then finds a suitable host and attaches to it. The larvae can survive more than 3 months without feeding. Once fully fed the larvae falls off and will moult to nymph on the ground in case of multiple host ticks or will start moulting to nymphs on the animal in case of single host ticks. The nymph has a scutum and four pairs of legs. But they will not possess the genital opening. The nymphs then moult to adult ticks either on host or from the ground then finds a suitable host for attachment. According to the length of the mouth parts the ticks have been grouped as brevirostrate (short) and longirostrate (elongated). Some of the common parasitic tick species prevalent in India along with their morphological features have been mentioned below.

Brevirostrate Ticks

Rhipicephalus sanguineus

Brown Dog Tick

They have short mouth parts. The head and mouth parts of ticks are together known as Basis capitulum. The ticks of the genus *Rhipicephalus* possess a hexagonal basis capitulum. Festoons are present posteriorly. Ist coxa is bifid. The inner margin of anal plate is straight in males.

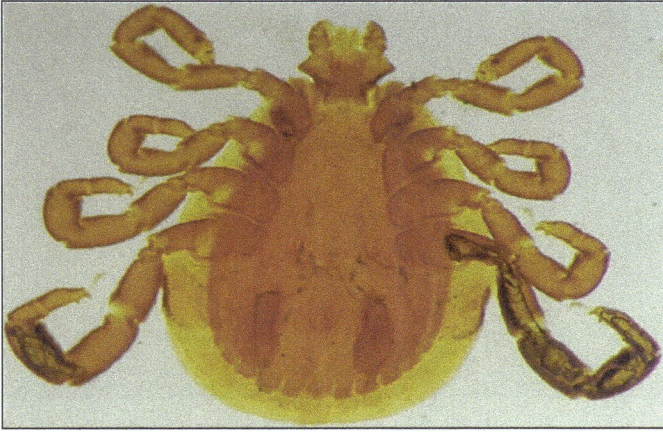

Figure 11: *Rhiphicephalus* **Species of Tick Observed under the Microscope.**

Rhipicephalus haemaphysaloides

The morphological features are similar to that of *Rhipicephalus sanguineus*. The inner margin of anal plate is curved in males.

Rhipicephalus (Boophilus) microplus

Tropical Cattle Tick

Previously these ticks were classified under the genus Boophilus, but recently due to the similarity in biochemical and molecular biological characters they are grouped in genus Rhipicephalus. They possess short mouth parts. Festoons are absent. Males have adanal shields and presence of a projection at the posterior margin of the body. The first coxa is bifid.

Rhipicephalus (Boophilus) annulatus

They closely resemble *R. (B). microplus* except for the posterior margin were they lack the projection.

Haemaphysalis anomala

Basis captulum dorsally wider than long. Second palpal segment is wider than the third. Lateral prolongation of the 2nd segment of the pedipalp extending beyond the basis capitulum. The mouth parts are short. Eyes are absent. First coxa have a pointed spine. Festoons are present. There are no adanal shields.

Haemaphysalis bispinosa

Similar to *Haemaphysalis anomala* except that 2nd and third palpal segment are equal in length. The spur on coxa I is bluntly pointed.

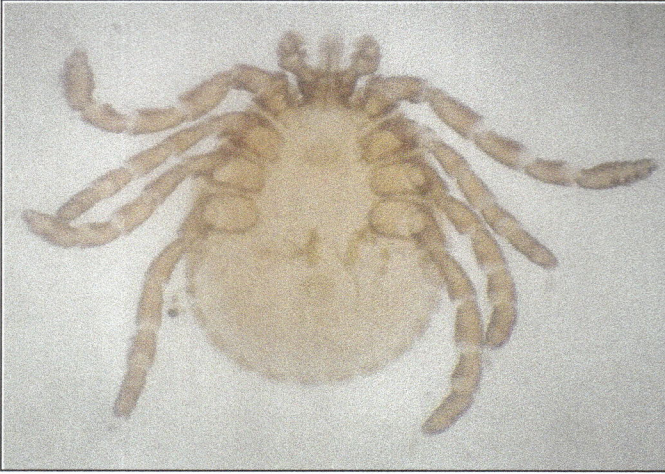

Figure 12: *Hemaphysalis* **Species of Tick Observed under the Microscope.**

Haemaphysalis intermedia

Basis capitulum is rectangular. The third palpal segment is longer than the second in males and in females it is comparatively short. Spur on coxa I is longer when compared to other coxae.

Longirostrate Ticks

Hyalomma anatolicum anatolicum

Bont Legged Tick

They are oval in shape. Mouth parts are long. Basis capitulum dorsally with slightly concave posterior margin and they are never angular. Basis capitulum does

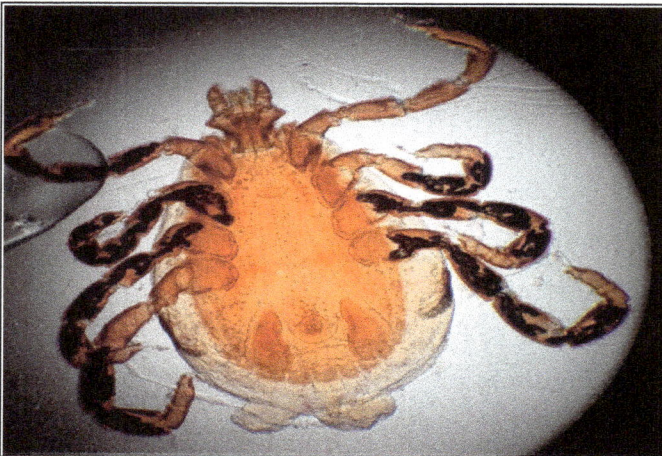

Figure 13: *Hyalomma* **Species of Tick Observed under the Microscope.**

not have lateral projections ventrally. The 2nd segment of the palp is as long as the 3ʳᵈ segment. The scutum is inornate. Coxa I deeply divided into narrow external spur and wider internal spur. Anal plates are well developed in males. In females the legs are not ringed with white pigment. Festoons are present, the central festoon is otherwise known as parma. There are grooves on the on the scutum. The lateral grooves will not reach the central third of the scutum. Postero median groove does not reach the parma.

Hyalomma dromedarii

Similar to *Hyalomma anatolicum anatolicum* except for the posteromedian groove, which will reach upto the parma. In females the legs are usually ringed with white pigment.

Hyalomma marginatum isaaci

Parma is absent. The leg segment has sharply defined rings on joints. The cervical grooves are deep. In females the scutum is dark brown in colour.

Hyalomina (Hyalomma) hussaini

Basis capituli ventrally possess lateral projections. Median and paramedian grooves are deep and distinct. Cervical grooves are distinct in case of females.

Amblyomma intergum

Body is round in shape. First and second palpal segments are almost equal in length. The 2nd segment of the palp is longer than the 3ʳᵈ segment. They have different pigmentation on the scutum so they are known as ornate ticks. Legs have rings of white pigment at the far ends of the segment. Coxa I with long sharply pointed spine like external spur and a short internal spur. Coxa II and III has only one spur in the form of a broad ridge. Anal plates may be present but usually small. Festoons are present.

Amblyomma testudinarium

Similar to *Amblyomma intergum*. Basis capitulum is rectangle shaped. Second palpal segment is longer than the first and third. All the four coxae are provided with a single spur, and the spur on fourth coxa is longest. The spur of coxa II and III are equal in length and they are shorter than the other two.

Testing of Acaricide Efficacy and Determination of Acaricidal Resistance

Different acaricides/insecticides are used against ectoparasites infesting animals. There are herbal and chemical acaricides and insecticides. The efficacy of newly introduced formulations of these drugs should be tested *invitro* before using it on the animals. The chemical acaricides face a major problem of resistance development in ticks because of the frequent and indiscriminate use. Whenever a newer compound/formulations are introduced in the market, it becomes imperative for a veterinarian to assess the efficacy of those compounds.

Resistance is usually first recognized as a failure of treatment to eliminate tick burdens from cattle. Although failure of treatment is often the result of incorrect preparation or application of acaricide, the persistence of ticks after frequent, correctly applied treatments indicates that acaricide resistance is likely. Because of the technically exacting requirements of the bioassays for resistance, very specific requirements exist with regard to the number, stage and age of the ticks and will vary according to the purpose of the test. Different stages of the tick like engorged females and adult males are collected from naturally infested dogs. In the laboratory, engorged female ticks collected are kept in petri dishes with a filter paper at the bottom in the desiccator containing saturated potassium chloride solution which provides a relative humidity of 80 per cent and temperature of 25°C (Sisodia *et al.*, 1986). Different developmental stages of ticks are obtained by rearing ticks on rabbits by using ear bag method. Numerous methods have been devised for detection of efficacy of acaricides/insecticides but they are laborious and time consuming. Hence, few simpler and quicker methods are discussed here.

1. Tea Bag Method (Gladney *et al.*, 1972)

Tea bags are prepared by using special types of paper called heat sealable rice paper having specification of 165 GSM supplied by the manufactures on large rolls. The 11cm width rolls is cut into 4cm wide strips from the roll folding them length wise and sealing them on two sides with a soldering iron rod to make a flat envelope (4 x 5.5cm) closed on 3 sides.

A known number of each developmental stages of tick such as eggs (100), larvae (50), nymphs (20), adult male ticks (10) and adult engorged females (5) are introduced separately into the tea bags which are sealed with a sealing rod. These tea bags are dipped in different concentrations of each acaricide with varying periods of time such as 50 sec for eggs, 3 sec for larvae and nymphs, 40 sec for adult male ticks and 50 sec for adult engorged females.

2. AIT Modified with a Discriminating Dose (AIT-DD)

The adult immersion test with a discriminating dose (AIT-DD) has been developed to provide a quicker and simpler test than the classical Drummond AIT. Using the AIT-DD, it is not necessary to weigh the eggs or to estimate the percentage hatch, allowing the test to be completed within 7 days rather than 4 to 5 weeks.

1. Dilute acaricides to the recommended discriminating doses.
2. Add 20 ml of the diluted acaricide to 100 ml plastic containers with screw-cap lids. Add 20 ml of water to another container as a control. Label the containers.
3. Add to each container a minimum of 10 healthy, clean, engorged female ticks taken from cattle within 48 h of the test.
4. Immerse ticks in acaricide solution for 30 minutes at about 25°C and shake containers gently.
5. After 30 minutes, pour off the acaricide solution into a safe storage container and dry the ticks gently on paper towelling.

6. Stick the ticks from one container, with ventral side up, onto double-sided sticky tape in a Petri dish.

7. Incubate the dishes in a larger polystyrene container at about 25 to 30°C for 7 days. Keep the container moist with damp paper or toweling. Do not shake the container as the egg batches from each tick have to be observed.

8. After 7 days count the number of ticks that have laid eggs. Ticks immersed in water only should have laid many eggs after 7 days. Ticks that have been treated with acaricide but still lay eggs are resistant. Ticks that have been treated with acaricide and do not lay eggs are susceptible.

The percentage resistance is calculated as: Resistance (per cent) = (Nt/Nw) × 100

where,

Nt = Number of treated ticks laying eggs

Nw = Number of untreated ticks laying eggs

In vitro Method of Evaluation of Insecticides for Fly Control

The effect of chemical compounds can be studied in *invitro* trials. Some of the insecticides commonly used against arthropod pests and currently available in the market include Cypermethrin, Fenvalerate, Propoxur.

Different concentrations of the insecticides are made *viz.*, for cypermethrin 0.7μg/cm², 1.5μg/cm² and 3.15μg/cm² concentration per cm² of filter paper as per for fenvalerate it is 1.5μg/cm², 3.15μg/cm² and 6.2μg/cm² of filter paper (Sheppard and Joyce 1992) and (Guglielmone *et al.*, 2001) for Propoxur 25mg, 50mg and 75mg.

The susceptibility of flies such as Haematobia, Stomoxys *etc.* can be assessed by using impregnated filter paper bioassays to evaluate the efficacy of above insecticides adapted from Sheppard and Hinkle 1987.

Steps

1. No.1 Whatman filter papers is laid into petridishes and treated with 1ml of desired concentrations of insecticides dissolved in acetone.

2. Then it is kept for three hours for drying.

3. The filter paper is kept in petridishes (9cm ×1.5cm) in which small holes are made at the top of the petridish to permit fly loading.

4. Then the flies are transferred in to it and observations are made.

5. Filter papers treated with 1ml acetone are used as controls.

6. After exposure to the insecticide, for two hours mortality is assessed. Percentage mortality data is analyzed by Abbott's formula.

$$\text{Efficacy per cent} = \frac{\text{Number of dead flies} - \text{Control mortality}}{\text{Number of used flies} - \text{Control mortality}} \times 100$$

The LC_{50} is determined by Probit analysis software.

Further Readings

1. Gladney W. J., Dawkins C.C. and Drummond R.O. (1972). Insecticides tested for control of nymphal brown dog ticks by the tea-bag technique. *J. Eco. Ent.* **65**:174-176.

2. Pradeep B.S., Renukaprasad C. and Placid E. D'Souza (2010). Evaluation of the commonly used acaricides against different stages of *Rhipicephalus sanguineus* by in vitro tests. *J. Vet. Para* 24(2): 185-188.

3. Pradeep B.S., Renukaprasad C. and Placid E. D'Souza (2012). Evaluation of the commonly used acaricides against different stages of the cattle tick *Boophilus microplus* by using different in vitro tests. *Indian J. Anim. Res.* 46(3): 248-252

4. Study on the bionomics and control of *Haematobia irritans* flies infesting Cattles-M.D.Bawer (2010). M.V.Sc thesis submitted to KVAFSU, Bidar- Unpublished.

Chapter 17

Geographical Information System (GIS) and its Applications in Veterinary Epidemiology

P. Krishnamoorthy

ICAR-National Institute of Veterinary Epidemiology and Disease Informatics (NIVEDI), Post Box No. 6450, Ramagondanahalli, Yelahanka, Bengaluru – 560 064, Karnataka

Geographic information systems (GIS) are "automated systems for the capture, storage, retrieval, analysis, and display of spatial data". A GIS is a constellation of computer hardware and software that integrates maps and graphics with a database related to a defined geographical space. The geographical data may be spatial or

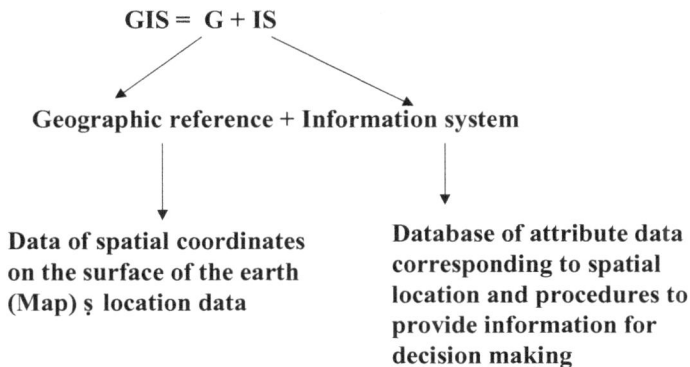

$$GIS = G + IS$$

Geographic reference + Information system

Data of spatial coordinates on the surface of the earth (Map) ş location data

Database of attribute data corresponding to spatial location and procedures to provide information for decision making

GIS = IS with geographically referenced data

descriptive in nature. A GIS can be defined as an integrated set of tools within an automated system capable of collecting, storing, handling, analyzing, and displaying geographically referenced information.

A GIS has several components, each with different functions, including the capability to:

- ☆ Digitize maps, which mean that the system captures spatial data for map preparation

- ☆ Store, handle, and integrate geographically referenced data from different sources, that is, it performs some functions of a database manager system;

- ☆ Retrieve or locate geographic data, which means that by locating points on a spatial surface, a number of attributes can be determined for that unit in the system;

- ☆ Produce various types of data analyses, including a capability for defining such conditions as adjacency, inclusion, and proximity;

- ☆ Produce output in several formats such as maps, graphs, and tables; and

- ☆ Produce high-quality thematic maps,

Since different output formats can be employed simultaneously and versatile editing tools are available. Some software packages-EpiMap and SiMap are two-have some of these capabilities, such as retrieving, storing, and displaying data through maps and may be used for basic GIS and epidemiological surveillance. If simultaneous management of different variables or databases is required, then more powerful computer programs are available. A GIS makes it possible to produce different types of analytical maps. One of them is the reference map, which shows the boundaries of certain areas and the location of different objects within them that are usually labeled. An example is a highway map with several types of roads, municipal boundaries, distances, towns, and other features. Due to their conceptual simplicity, superimposing layers of information, reference maps are attractive because they can be easily handled as a set of images. Thematic or choropleth maps have areas that are colored or marked in accordance with a key so that the color or marking reflects the intensity of a mapped variable. Examples of these types of maps include among others: the area map, which shows a phenomenon according to a particular territory; the symbol map, which shows scattered objects in relation to points on the map; the isoarithmic or isoline map, which shows phenomena with uniform changes in a pattern of uninterrupted diffusion; the dotdensity map, which shows the occurrence of a phenomenon with nonuniform distribution; the cartodiagram in which the size of territorial units represents the magnitude of a phenomenon. A GIS makes it possible to perform other operations that are valuable in decision analysis and decision-making: redistricting of boundaries, defining of buffer areas or buffering, and determining the distance between objects. In redistricting, the boundaries of one territory can be modified or joined to those of another in order to form a new territory including in these operations the sum of the values of their attributes into a single unit. Buffering allows contiguous or non-contiguous territories or objects of different shapes and dimensions to be selected in order to form a virtual region or area without having to modify boundaries. Both redistricting and buffering capture the information on attributes of an area or region so that they can be managed or analyzed. Distance determination makes it possible to calculate the real distance between two or more points on a map or the area of a territory. Finally, some GIS packages have the ability to process images such as aerial or satellite photographs, thereby offering continuous and systematic coverage of different types of information within large geographical tracts.

Data and Files Required for a GIS and their Sources

There are essentially two types of data used in a geographical information system: cartographic data and descriptive or attribute data. Cartographic data provide a spatial or geographical reference for an object, whereas attribute information indicates the characteristics of the object. In general, a GIS contains four types of information and computer files: geographic, map, attribute, and data-point files. Geographic files are the heart of a GIS; they contain the data, including the coordinates defining each unit that are going to be mapped. The map files contain information on the names of geographical files and other related files forming the GIS; *e.g.*, names or labels, coverage, colors, map scale, and lines. Attribute files are rectangular data files whose columns list variables and whose rows correspond to individual cases or geographical points. Finally, data-point files are those produced by linking interfacing attribute files and geographic files through a process called geocoding, using an identifier. If such a map is not available, the clear alternative is to prepare a map independently. This can be done through one of three methods: electronic digitizing, data conversion, or the use of global positioning systems (GPS). Digitizing consists of manually transferring maps in hardcopy to an electronic format. This method requires a digitizing tablet to place points on a map, which are subsequently joined by lines. In contrast to points situated with a mouse, which only supply their relative position on a plane, the absolute position is provided for the point entered with a digitizing tablet, and the defined point will always have the same position of coordinates available, so distances can also be determined. Alternatively, scanners may be employed to reproduce hardcopy maps, although expensive precision equipment is required to transform images to vector formats that can be handled by the GIS. As might be expected, preparation of maps with these procedures requires a considerable time investment, and their quality depends on the accuracy of source maps and the skills of the technician. Data conversion is done through the selection of control points on maps by their known coordinates for latitude and longitude; the values are then entered for a number of points whose coordinates have been defined through formulas. In this case as well, precision in making calculations and quality of the source maps for the control points are essential. Finally, the global positioning system (GPS) is used to find a location in the field through radio transmission to satellites, which provide the coordinates for the point of transmission. Each option has a different level of precision and cost, which means the decision on what to use must take account of needs and available resources.

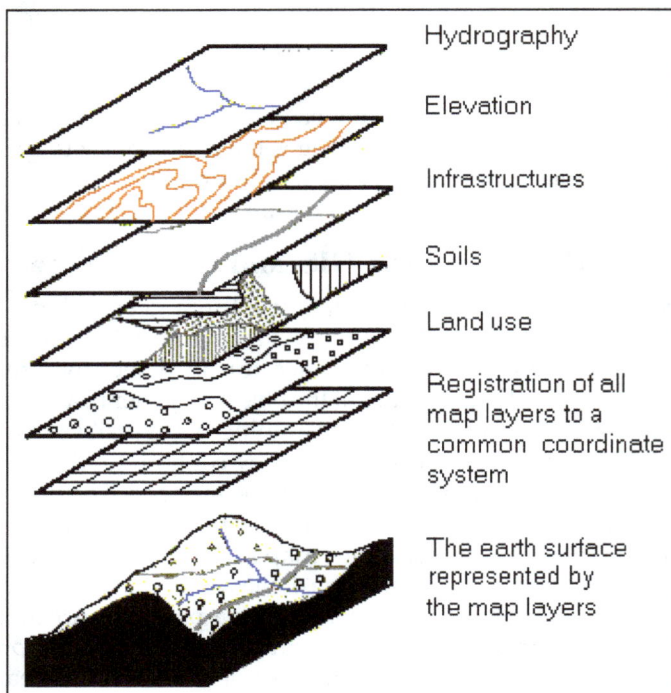

Hydrography

Elevation

Infrastructures

Soils

Land use

Registration of all map layers to a common coordinate system

The earth surface represented by the map layers

Map Layer Overlay

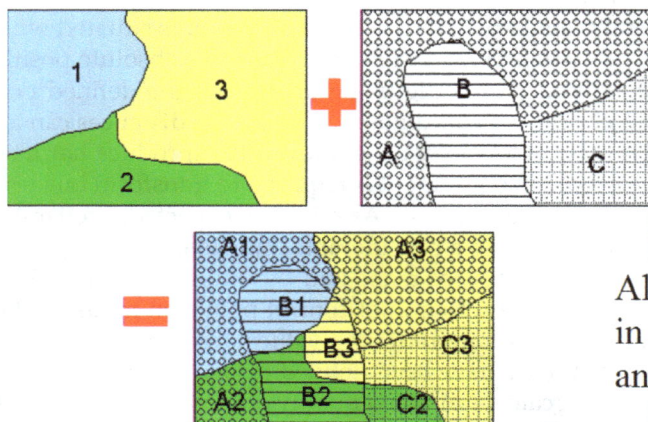

All layers must be in same projection and scale

Overlay generates homogenous units – eg. agroecozones

Source: FAO

Use of GIS in Epidemiology

GIS use in the field of public health is quite new. The development of these systems gained momentum in other areas such as marketing, transportation, law enforcement, and monitoring geological and climatic phenomena around the world. GIS can be applied in Epidemiology (Epi-GIS), for different aspects most of which are interconnected. Some of the most common uses are the determination of the health situation in an area, generation and analysis of research hypotheses, identification of high-risk health groups, planning and programming of activities, and monitoring and evaluation of interventions.

Recording and Reporting Disease Information

GIS can be used to produce maps of disease incidence, prevalence, mortality, morbidity on farm, region, or national levels. The information is more easily understood when visualized on a map. Because information on diseases often tends to be aggregated (from information on each individual herd to municipality or county level) the information loses some of its value. If the information is mapped at the farm level, only small parts of a region can be visualized at the same time.

Epidemic Emergency

In case of an outbreak of an infectious disease, GIS can provide an excellent tool for identifying the location of the case farm and all farms at risk within a specified area of the outbreak. Buffer zones can be drawn around those farms and with a link to tables of the addresses of the farms at risk; the farms can be informed within a short time after a notified outbreak. Buffer zones can also be generated around other risk areas or point sources, such as roads where infected cattle have been driven or around market places. Further, the maps can assist the field veterinarians to plan their work in the current situation, and for the veterinary authorities in how to handle a potential outbreak.

Analysis of Clustering of Diseases

To analyse whether a disease is clustered in space, time or in time and space other programs still have to be used because this is not yet a standard tool in the available GIS-packages. The visualisation of the disease rates on digital maps can be misleading because the eye tends to interpret point patterns as clusters more often than what is real. Therefore, a cluster analysis should be carried out for an objective evaluation of the reported disease cases. The results of some of the cluster analyses can, thereafter, be imported into a GIS to visualise the location of clusters or cluster areas.

Model Disease Spread

Simulation models using programmes packages as @Risk (Palisade Corporation, Newfield, NY, USA) can be integrated within a GIS. Such simulation models can incorporate farm information such as herd size, production type as well as spatial factors like distance to the source of outbreak, population density and climate conditions, vegetation and landscape, all of which have been defined as risk factors for the spread of the modelled disease. Sanson, (1994) has developed a model of a potential outbreak of foot and mouth disease in New Zealand.

Planning Disease Control Strategies

The neighbourhood analysis function can be used to identify all adjacent farms to an infected farm. It is a function that identifies all adjacent features with a certain criteria to a particular feature. Contact patterns such as common use of grasslands or sources of purchasing *etc.* could be visualised with a so-called spider diagram. This could provide insight into the possibility of transmission of infectious diseases between herds. In the planning of eradication of diseases, GIS has the possibility to perform overlay analysis to find high or low risk areas for diseases which depend on geographical features or conditions related to the geography. Studies of trypanosomiasis and theileriosis are just some examples of how to use GIS to plan eradication of diseases depending on habitats of vectors or wild animal population. GIS could also be used to find areas with a low density of other farms or risk areas of diseases as shown by Staubach *et al.* (1998) in case of Echinococcus multilocularis in foxes. A GIS provides significant added value to current routine data that is usually taken into low consideration for either epidemiological or management purposes in veterinary medicine. A GIS considerably increases the efficacy of communication. Management and veterinary service tasks and resources during emergency can be improved with the use of GIS. Description of geographical disease dynamics over time, of risk factors due to spatial relationships as well as the drawing of risk and damage maps becomes feasible. The deficiencies in a surveillance system also become more obvious and as a by-product of introduction of GIS, the system of collecting, storing and managing data can be improved.

GIS will find a variety of applications in Veterinary public health, particularly for diseases where environment or habitat factors influence disease occurrence. Rabies is one obvious example where the technique has particular application, but there are numerous examples among other diseases in various countries. GIS will mainly be adopted first in research on zoonoses, but will gradually be adopted for disease control. Most of the management applications of GIS will be in form of integrated decision support systems which make field disease control programs more effective and target them more precisely to control needs.

Further Readings

1. Aronoff, S. (1991). Geographic Information Systems: A management Perspective, WDL Publications, canada.

2. ESRI (1990). Understanding GIS.

3. FAO : http://www.fao.org/sd/eidirect/gis/EIgis000.htm

4. Heywood I, Cornelius S.,and Carver, S. (1998). An Introduction to Geographical Information Systems, Longman pub., 279 pp.

5. Longley, P.A., Goodchild, M.F., Maguire, D.J. and Rhind, D.W (eds) (1999). Geographic Information Systems, Volumes 1 and 2, Wiley pub.

6. http://www.colorado.edu/geography/gcraft/notes

Chapter 18

Spatial Epidemiology: An Introduction

Divakar Hemadri

ICAR-National Institute of Veterinary Epidemiology and Disease Informatics (NIVEDI), Post Box No. 6450, Ramagondanahalli, Yelahanka, Bengaluru – 560 064, Karnataka

Spatial Epidemiology

Spatial epidemiology is the description and analysis of geographic variations in disease with respect to demographic, environmental, behavioral, socioeconomic, genetic, and infectious risk factors

Why to Analyse Disease Data Spatially

It may be noted that many diseases are spatially constrained; for example, vector-borne and zoonotic diseases occur where and when vectors, animal hosts, pathogens and susceptible human populations overlap. Vectors, pathogens and animal populations are unevenly distributed in space and time and as a result risk for exposure to vectorborne diseases is spatially heterogeneous. Therefore, spatial models for the study and management of vector-borne disease risk have become common with the development of digitally encoded environmental data and computational tools such as geographical information systems (GIS). It is estimated that over 90 per cent of health data (animal and human) has a spatial or geographical component.

- ☆ Variations in disease outbreaks are better understood if neighbouring farm networks are taken into account?
- ☆ geography can also be used as a proxy

    e.g., measuring the distribution of outbreaks against vaccination activity, i.e "is there more FMD in non-vaccinated areas";

☆ and finally geography is a very useful framework for communication for example "how does the livestock health in Mizoram compare to Sikkim is more easily understandable when mapped

What do you Require to do Spataial Analysis

☆ Disease data

        Time (if available datewise very good)

        No of cases (no. affected)

        Total population

        No of deaths

☆ Demographic Data

        Specieswise data

☆ Environmental Data

        Rainfall

        Temperature

        Wind speed

        Wind direction

        Relative humidity

        Vector Data

☆ Socio-economic Data

☆ Land Cover and Land Use Data

☆ Soil Data

☆ Digital Maps

        Lat Long

☆ Real-time satellite images

☆ Finally, skill and will

What can be Achieved in Spatial Epidemiology

Disease Mapping

Disease mapping is a eld that concentrates on the spatial variation in the risk of disease. Basic map styles commonly used for disease mapping include Dot maps, Choropleth maps, Isopleth maps.

Dot maps, are suitable for presenting point data referenced in two-dimensional coordinate space, such as the locations of disease events.

Choropleth maps are tremendously common and useful. These use some existing system of boundaries (countries, states, counties, voting districts, *etc.*). In choropleth maps, data is grouped into or more levels or classes using slicing values. These maps show spatial variation of one or two variables at a time by using color, shades of grey and/or patterns

Isopleth maps are especially well fitted for inspecting continuously varying phenomena, such as temperature, rainfall *etc.* These maps feature continuously varying color values basically by a line on a map that connects points of equal value.

Geographic Correlation Studies

These look at correlations between variables. For example, a study may investigate the occurrence of meningococcal infection. In doing this it might correlate the economical status and personal hygiene of people. One would expect that as level of infection to be more among economically weaker class. Some studies may focus on habitat mapping of a particular species of insect based on the data obtained from a small survey. Another example of geographical correlation studies is relating human taeniasis infection with heavily infected cysticercotic pigs.

The Assessment of Risk in Relation to a Point or Line-Source

Point and line-source studies assume a risk source that has the shape of a point or a line, such as a chimney or an electrical wire. Highly localized studies are conducted in order to discover possible increases in ill-health due to increased exposure from these specic types of sources.

Cluster Detection and Disease Clustering

Cluster detection is carried out in order to detect raised levels of incidence of disease. If disease cases seem to form non-random patterns, that is, clusters, then there is reason to suspect that the underlying effect is non-random. It can provide information on the etiological background of the disease. A spatial disease cluster may be defined as an area with an unusually elevated disease incidence rate. The identification of a cluster of disease can help epidemiologists determining putative environmental risk factors and lead to improved understanding of etiology.

Commonly Encountered P:roblems in Spatial Epidemiological Studies

☆ Non availability of good quality of data which may lead to Garbage in = Garbage out kind of situation.

☆ Georeferencing of attribute data

☆ Government data rich but information poor

☆ Lag time between environmental exposure and presentation

☆ Biological plausibility – does it make sense (critical thinking skills)

☆ Spatial data is expensive

☆ Spatial data must be accurate and up to date

☆ Complexity of analysis - requires training

☆ Complexity of activity – multiple exposures points

☆ Interpretation - ecological fallacy, aggregating data

Summary

☆ Spatial epidemiology is the study of the spatial patterns, processes nd determinants of health and disease

☆ Spatial epidemiological methods use GIS and spatial based analytical tools

☆ A GIS can place data in an environmental context – but don't overlook human input

Chapter 19

Animal Quarantine and Certification Services in India: An Overview

Jimlee Sharma

Animal Quarantine and Certification Service,
Kempegowda International Airport, Devanahalli, Karnataka

With the increase of international trade and travel, every country is becoming more and more exposed to the danger of introduction of known and unknown transmissible diseases which have the potential for very serious and rapid spread, irrespective of national borders, serious socio-economic or public health consequence and major importance in the international trade of animal and animal products. Some of those serious diseases of livestock are present in other countries but do not prevail in India.

Therefore, it became necessary to prevent the entry of any exotic disease through international trade and travel in to India and to ensure the health and safety of the animal and human life.

Keeping this in view, Government of India initiated a central sector scheme namely "Animal Quarantine and Certification Services" (AQCS) during the Fourth Five Year Plan (1969-70) under which four Animal Quarantine stations were set up at Delhi, Chennai, Kolkata and Mumbai.Thereafter in the year 2009,two new stations at Hyderabad and Bangalore were also notified as Quarantine Stations and both the stations are under construction with only certain livestock and products being allowed to be imported through these ports. The responsibility of preventing ingress of exotic diseases and thereby safeguarding the health of country's livestock population lies solely with the Animal Quarantine and Certification services.

Purpose

The major objective of the Animal Quarantine and Certification Services is to prevent ingress of livestock and poultry diseases exotic to India and issue export certificate of live animals as per the international requirements.

Scheme on Animal Quarantine and Certification Services

The Animal Quarantine and Certification Services activities are being performed by the Regional/Quarantine Officers at the six AQCS Stations located one each at the six major International ports at Delhi, Mumbai, Chennai, Hyderabad, Bangalore and Kolkata. These stations are functioning under the control of Department of Animal Husbandry and Dairying, Ministry of Agriculture, New Delhi.

The Animal Quarantine and Certification Services in India have been taking prompt measures to protect the country from the ingress of any exotic animal diseases. As soon as the presence of a new disease is noticed in a particular country, immediate action is taken, prohibiting the import of susceptible species of animals and their products from that country.

The responsibility for implementation of import protocols, supervision of importations, extending quarantine facilities and procedures remain with Animal Quarantine and Certification Services. The supervision of imported commodities involves surveillance, monitoring, direct inspection/examination; quarantine, testing if necessary and certification and clearance at port of entry *i.e.* Delhi, Kolkata, Mumbai Chennai,Hyderabad and Bangalore. These functions contribute in managing the risk of importations.

This programme also envisages provision of an internationally acceptable certification services for the export of animal and animal products, comply with importing country's health requirements or the health regulations prescribed in the Terrestrial Animal Health Code, O.*I.E.*

General Obligations in International Trade and Quarantine Interventions

International trade in animal and animal products depends on a combination of factors, which should be taken into account to ensure unimpeded trade, without incurring unacceptable risks to human and animal health.

Because of the likely variations in animal health situations, the O.I.E Terrestrial Animal Health Code offers various options. The animal health situation in the exporting country, in the transit country or countries and in the importing country should be considered before determining the requirements, which have to be met for trade. To maximize harmonization of the sanitary aspects of international trade, Veterinary Administrations should base their import requirements on the OIE standards, guidelines and recommendations.

The Animal Quarantine Regulation in India

Importation of Livestock and Livestock products are regulated by the Livestock

Importation Act, 1898 (Act No. 9 of 1898) and as amended by the Livestock Importation (Amendment) Act, 2001 (28 of 2001) (Annexure-II) and as notified in the official Gazette/official orders from time to time.

Functions of Animal Quarantine and Certification Services in India

Entry of any livestock or livestock product is regulated by the Livestock Importation Act, 1898 as amended in 2001. These importations are allowed subject to fulfillment of health/quarantine requirements specified by the Government of India that are developed depending upon the disease status of the exporting country and the species of Livestock/type of product to be imported.

☆ Implementation of various provisions of Livestock Importation Act, 1898 (as amended in 2001).

☆ Quarantine/Testing of imported livestock and livestock products.

☆ Export certification of Livestock/Livestock Products as per the requirements of the importing country and as prescribed in the Terrestrial Animal Health Code, *O.I.E.* and in consultation with Export Inspection Council (EIC) in the areas not covered under EIC.

Index

www.ingramcontent.com/pod-product-compliance
Lightning Source LLC
Chambersburg PA
CBHW060249230326
41458CB00094B/1585